THE DENTAL PRACTICE "JUGGLERS"
The Ultimate Practice Manager's Guide

Ashley Latter
and
Alistair Mann

authorHOUSE®

AuthorHouse™ UK
1663 Liberty Drive
Bloomington, IN 47403 USA
www.authorhouse.co.uk
Phone: 0800 047 8203 (Domestic TFN)
+44 1908 723714 (International)

© 2019 Ashley Latter and Alistair Mann. All rights reserved.

No part of this book may be reproduced, stored in a retrieval system, or transmitted by any means without the written permission of the author.

Published by AuthorHouse 09/12/2019

ISBN: 978-1-7283-9039-0 (sc)
ISBN: 978-1-7283-9038-3 (e)

Print information available on the last page.

Any people depicted in stock imagery provided by Getty Images are models, and such images are being used for illustrative purposes only. Certain stock imagery © Getty Images.

This book is printed on acid-free paper.

Because of the dynamic nature of the Internet, any web addresses or links contained in this book may have changed since publication and may no longer be valid. The views expressed in this work are solely those of the author and do not necessarily reflect the views of the publisher, and the publisher hereby disclaims any responsibility for them.

Contents

Thank You ix

Chapter 1: Practice Managers - The Practice "Jugglers" 1
Chapter 2: Presenting Change and Effective
 Communication 22
Chapter 3: Productive Meetings 38
Chapter 4: Staff Motivation 49
Chapter 5: Coaching, Mentoring and Feedback 58
Chapter 6: Delegation 74
Chapter 7: Staff Underperformance 89
Chapter 8: Managing Upwards 95
Chapter 9: Time Management 106

Epilogue 119
Practice Managers Club 125

Ashley Latter is synonymous with the dental profession having coached almost 20,000 delegates in a phenomenal career spanning more than 20 years. His legendary two day "Ethical Sales & Communication" programme has now conquered the globe, reaching countries like Canada, USA, Australia and India.

He's now delivered over 28,000 hours of business coaching to the dental industry and has gained a reputation as being the best around at getting dentists, orthodontists and their teams to effectively communicate with their patients and thereby create the perfect patient journey.

Married to Graziella, with two children Enrica and Martina, he loves nothing better than walking with them in the Lake District, cycling and watching his beloved Manchester United.

Author of the hugely successful books 'Don't wait for the tooth fairy', and "You are worth it", Ashley now adds a third must-have publication to his growing portfolio.

Alistair is a well–respected specialist course presenter on management and leadership. Having trained as an adult education coach in 2006, he has been offering delegates right across the employment spectrum his expertise ever since and has worked with a number of internationally renowned companies.

Educated at Manchester Grammar School, he studied Journalism at UCLAN, before subsequently working for ITV for more than 16 years, fulfilling a variety of roles including as a producer, presenter and commentator. It was those skills in particular that have enabled him to develop many of the programmes he currently successfully delivers, offering a unique insight into improving self-confidence and enhancing assertive leadership.

A professional sports broadcaster he has presented and commentated all over the world, with the BBC, BT Sport, ITV and Sky Sports all on his impressive CV, as well as three National RTS Television Awards and a BT Sports Journalist of the year award, in recognition of his successful career to date.

Married to Lissa, they have one son (Ethan), one dog (Stewie) and one cat (Maggie), meaning his spare time is usually split between Dad's taxi service and dog walking duties!

Alistair and Ashley have worked together since 2013, delivering courses to hundreds of delegates across the UK and Ireland and continue to receive outstanding reviews for their distinctive style of coaching. This book is their second collaboration, with Alistair having also edited Ashley's "You are Worth It" in 2014.

Thank You

This book became a reality after having spent many pleasurable hours working with some of the most talented professionals we've ever had the privilege of coaching. In our experience, almost without exception, practice managers have an eagerness to make themselves the very best they can be and that willingness to take on new ideas has always marked them out as ideal delegates to coach. Without their contributions over the past few years this book would not have been possible.

In particular we'd like to thank: Susie Anderson-Sharkey, Lorraine Browne, Caroline Burnett, Jennifer Hopper and Kerry Scott.

CHAPTER 1

Practice Managers - The Practice "Jugglers"

Welcome to the world of practice management. If you are new to it – good luck; if you're a veteran – congratulations! Either way, you are a special person with an amazing array of talents.

The first thing to establish is that a dental practice is a business and as such you need to be aware, if you weren't already, that you are a business manager. Here's how one business recruitment magazine describes this integral role:

"Business managers are responsible for overseeing and supervising a company's activities and employees. Small businesses rely on the business manager to keep workers aligned with the goals of the company. Business managers report to top executives in a larger organization, but in a small company, the manager might either own the company or report directly to the owner."

Whether this sounds like you or not, one thing which we are sure about is that you will be a very busy individual, with a feeling that every aspect of the practice is your responsibility, from the replenishing of toilet paper in the men's loos, right through to the staff rotas! Throw in some additional specific tasks unique to dentistry, like CQC and compliance and its clear why this role is seen as one of the most complex and challenging roles in business. That said, with such a variety of different responsibilities, this is also why it is viewed as one of the most satisfying careers for a manager in the entire industrial market place.

We've been coaching practice managers (PMs) for many years and if there's one thing we've found as a common trait among every single one of them, it is their core desire to make the practice a success. PMs may not be the owners but they treat their practices as if they were, with the same passion and commitment as the owners themselves; what we have also found, all too often, is that this enviable level of professionalism leads them to charge from one task to another, stretching even their seemingly endless supply of enthusiasm to breaking point.

The very best PMs we have dealt with, have an incredible ability to seamlessly move from one task to another, with aplomb. One moment they can be advising a staff member on reception, the next they can be negotiating a new price with a supplier; we've seen a PM escort an elderly patient to their car, then five minutes later chair a meeting, devising a complex new marketing strategy; each task carried out to the maximum and with hardly a break in their stride; done with all the dexterity and panache of a skilled juggler.

So how can a PM become such a highly skilled "juggler"? How do they prevent every single "ball" in the practice from crashing to the ground? How do they become the most valuable "performer" in the dental practice "circus"? Well, to keep this analogy going for just one more sentence, "roll up, roll up and welcome to our guide to the greatest show on earth", as we guide you through the secrets of how to keep all those balls in the air!

THE JOURNEY TO PRACTICE MANAGER

We will begin this journey by analysing yours and establishing how you became a PM in the first place. There are naturally two different routes: one is a promotion from within the existing staff at a practice; the other is an outside appointment and while both ultimately share common challenges, each journey to that point is unique. It is important therefore to establish and distinguish these two very different backgrounds and the separate challenges they subsequently create.

PMs recruited from outside

A PM who is recruited from outside the practice will initially have a very different set of hurdles to negotiate. For a start of course, unlike an internally promoted appointee, the staff are unlikely to know anything about you, which will, at first, lead to a period of tentative and largely superficial meet and greets.

We are all aware of the significance of first impressions and in these circumstances, making a successful start can certainly help in the process of building trust and earning respect. While it is a gross exaggeration to suggest that these early meetings are pivotal in establishing yourself among your new colleagues, it is still important that you attempt to do what you can to make them as impactful as possible; and to that end there are a number of things you can do.

A little homework is a useful thing. While you don't want to spook anybody, there is no harm in trying to find out some information about your new employees. Ask the practice owners for a brief potted history of each of them and make a note of anything significant.

There could be an employee who is getting married this year, or one who has recently become a grandparent; perhaps there is someone who has recently returned from an exotic holiday or has just given up smoking; a friendly congratulatory statement from a newly recruited PM, can certainly make a difference as staff begin to formulate their opinion of you.

Equally, it can be important to be aware of any negative issues which may affect the mood of an individual when you first say hello. There are a number of factors which will have a significant impact on their demeanour; there could be an employee who has recently suffered a family bereavement or has a relative who is currently hospitalised; becoming aware of this, can save you from saying something, which could be interpreted as being insensitive.

Additionally, it can also be useful to find out about employees who have been having work-related issues; but while it may be helpful to know for example, about a staff member who you beat to the job, at this early stage, it is equally important not to form any opinions before you've met them. You wouldn't want an employee to have preconceived ideas about you, so it is important that you haven't already made up your mind up about them. In the workplace, people can surprise you and as a manager, being open minded, is a quality which shouldn't be overlooked.

The title of PM carries with it a sense of importance and responsibility and as such appearance is another significant factor of which to be aware. Leaders should always be smart and professional, so even if you're a jeans and t-shirt kind of person, you should consider abandoning this casual look in favour of more suitable attire. While nobody should have to try to be something they are not, dentistry naturally has to adhere to the principles of clinical hygiene, so to be clean and well-presented is a must for a new PM from the outset.

Over the years we've met PMs whose very first aim on being appointed was to change the dress code at their new practice – that process can begin on day one, by they themselves demonstrating what they feel is appropriate work wear.

Another aspect to consider when it comes to making a first impression is time keeping. PMs have to be seen to be the example setters for the entire staff, so if you want your team to be punctual, then so should you be. While punctuality should be consistently maintained to be impactful in the long term, new PMs should actually endeavour to arrive early from day one, to rule out any chance of a late train or a broken down car preventing a timely arrival. The last thing a new PM wants is to play catch up on their first day at the practice, so why not build in a little extra time for a coffee, ahead of the day's travails.

Pre-surgery team meetings are becoming more prevalent at UK practices, so a confident PM may even want to introduce the concept from the outset, by requesting a get together on their first morning, in order to introduce themselves, formally, to their new team. If the practice you are joining already holds these early morning meets, then request that the main item on the agenda is your introduction – if the practice doesn't hold them and you want to make a bold statement, requesting that staff begin their day 15 minutes earlier than they are used to, will certainly let your new team know, that you mean business!

One thing which managers tend to neglect in their first few days at a new practice is the importance of listening carefully to what is being said to them. This applies to patients and staff alike. With so much going on as they familiarise themselves with their new job, PMs are so busy trying to make a good impression, that they don't realise that others are trying to do the same with them!

It is essential, therefore, that you are attentive to what's being pointed out and that you respond appropriately to what's being communicated. One sure-fire way of making a bad impression, is to mishear what's being said to you due to impatience, or diverting your attention elsewhere. Concentrated listening is a sign that you are interested and by being interested, it demonstrates that you care.

That concept of demonstrating care through attentive listening should extend to another of the senses – by maintaining eye contact with your new colleagues as you are first introduced. Eye contact is a very powerful tool in creating a good impression and has many powerful connotations beyond simply showing that you are genuinely interested.

Maintaining eye-contact gives off a feeling of warmth, while conversely, diverting your gaze elsewhere gives off the negative signal of appearing to be aloof. There's evidence to suggest that looking sincerely at someone while they speak, actually promotes a lengthier and invariably more meaningful conversation – this is much more likely to create an environment that will allow rapport to develop.

Eye contact also helps to build trust and demonstrates a sense of respect to others. Looking directly at someone suggests an equality and even if you are chatting with a subordinate over whom you will ultimately be presiding, this sense of respect, points to a fair minded leader, whose judgements are more likely to be appropriate.

Of course, this important trait shouldn't be exclusively reserved for first meetings and a continued use of eye contact throughout your managerial career, will convey a sense of understanding and empathy, which will maintain your position as a just leader.

While a new PM sets about making a good first impression, it is useful to take a momentary step back, to ponder why you have been brought into the practice in the first place. The most obvious starting point is of course that there was a vacancy but it's important for a new PM to ascertain why the vacancy occurred in the first place.

It is likely that during the hiring process a practice owner will have told you what happened to your predecessor but if it hasn't been explained, you are perfectly entitled to satisfy your curiosity, by finding out the reason. In truth it is a significant first step for any new recruit and a perfectly legitimate question to ask your new employer.

There are a variety of reasons why a vacancy existed prior to your deployment and each carries a different message to the new recruit. If your predecessor retired after decades of loyal service, there is a good chance that the staff they leave behind will have a sense of disappointment that their long-time colleague has gone and a real concern that you are going to change the entire dynamic of the practice, after years of continuity. Contrast that with a predecessor who left after a series of disputes and fall-outs and you will have an entirely different approach in mind for your new role.

In our experience, a new PM is often brought in by a new practice owner. Principal dentists who buy out a previous owner, will often feel that the best way to move on from his/her predecessor is to bring in new or additional staff, particularly at senior level. This is commonly the case when the previous owner has opted for retirement, with the new owner keen to stamp their own image on their new premises. Once again this should send out an entirely different message to the new PM about the way in which to approach their role.

Having established the reason why you've been brought in and consequently the way in which you need to tackle your new job, the next aspect to think about, is why you were recruited from outside the practice, rather than the vacancy being filled from within. The most obvious reason is that there weren't any suitable candidates at the practice, so there will have been little choice other than to look outside.

In our experience, however, the usual reason an outside candidate is brought in, is that a practice owner feels that an outsider will bring with them a whole new perspective to the business. In most industries, this has been a common policy of owners as they seek to move it forward or in another direction; as dentistry has been leaning towards private practice and away from the NHS, so the need to bring in an outside view has become more prevalent.

Business management is a most desirable skillset and the vast array of different assets which a shrewd manager possesses, allows them to transfer from one business to another with ease. In effect, the desirable qualities of a manager are what is important and not their knowledge of a particular industry. Principal dentists have quickly realised that this is the case and when a suitable candidate is not apparent within their practice, they are extremely comfortable in looking outside the dental profession, to find their new PM.

Over the years we've worked with PMs who have previously been employed across a raft of different genres – education, travel, mobile phone networks, even the military – and rather than this being seen as a negative, it has actually been viewed as quite the opposite, by a practice owner seeking an entirely fresh approach.

We recently worked with a PM on our practice manager's club year-long programme, who had previously been employed by a major tour operator. This is what she had to say about her own transition from a completely different field:

"My role has always been clearly defined. I am, in many ways detached from the dentistry. I leave that to the principal and the clinicians.

My strength I feel, is that I manage the practice from a different angle –from the experience I got from being an operations manager at a major tour operator, which gave me a view from a service perspective. On the basis that we are private, that works really well.

For example, I manage the dentists and the nurses in terms of the materials they need ordering but I'm not involved myself because of my lack of dental knowledge.

The principal has changed from the one who initially recruited me. The previous one, in terms of managing staff, managing patients and day to day work, could see that there were skills that they hadn't had previously at the practice.

His theory was that the majority of dental practices recruit from within; it tends to be a nurse, somebody that has worked their way up the ladder. That's great in terms of providing dental experience and knowledge but he wanted something different.

I think he felt that while you have technicians, hygienists and so on, they can tick these boxes but you then need someone who can then think outside the box in terms of the business and to manage it from a service orientated angle. And he saw that in me.

Initially I worked on reception, which is different in some respects but when I worked at the tour operator, at first I worked on the telephone there. It was like being in sales, converting each call into a booking. I found I could adapt that skill to the role on reception, so that every time the phone rang I could pin them down and get them to book in as a patient, before finally converting them to us on a full time basis.

At first, I admit I was concerned – concerned if I could adapt – but I soon realised I could smoothly use my experience to another profession.

When I was first made up to PM from reception, the dentist wasn't sure that I was going to be right for the position as I'd been working part time and he hadn't seen enough of me. But once we started to work together, we found we worked really well as a team. We went through a number of issues at first but I know now I have his full support. If he felt that I had made a wrong decision, he would tell me, but he would still support me.

I didn't at all feel that I was out of my depth due to my lack of dentistry knowledge. I knew I could handle it, as I knew that I could find out the answers to difficult questions. I've always been able to talk through things with team members and even when I talk to new recruits now, I explain to them my journey and the fact that from a clinical point of view, I don't necessarily have all the answers.

The fact is that I have the team around me to be able to find out all the answers. I'm only as good as the people I work with and actually when we work together, we are really good at what we do.

I'm lucky that I work in a practice where the dentists are very good at what they do, the hygienists are very good at what they do and the services we provide are second to none; we rarely have many complaints. The only real issues that I've had to face or address, I've always been able to deal with quite confidently, through my previous managerial experience.

When I was at the tour operator, I was the operations manager and I dealt with everything negative that could impact a client's holiday before they departed and whilst they were away. I knew how to turn that negative into a positive. The tour operator gave me such good training. They had an in-house training team where they invested huge amounts of time and effort into the service you provide as a tour operator. It meant that I was able to adjust and take those skills into dentistry."

It's vitally important to point out at this juncture, that this has, in no way, reduced the number of PMs who have been sourced from within the existing dental routes. In the past, PMs would largely be promoted, having previously served as dental nurses, receptionists, hygienists and so on; this is still the case and will continue to be so going forward. However, as the number of practices which are converting to private dentistry increases, so too has the demand for managers with

management experience, as owners deem it increasingly necessary to have more complex business models.

PMS WHO ARE PROMOTED FROM WITHIN.

Though there are of course many similar emotions which any new appointee will be feeling, a PM who has been promoted to the role, will face a series of unique initial challenges to that of an outsider, as they embark on this new stage of their career; most significantly, the feeling of stepping upwards from an equal, to a leader.

Perhaps the greatest challenge that a newly promoted PM will face, is how to command the respect of those who previously considered themselves your peers. There has to be an understanding that this is not something that you can hurry. It has to evolve naturally and you certainly can't accelerate it, no matter how much you would like to. The promotion in itself, doesn't automatically guarantee respect.

The best way to begin this process, is by carrying out your new duties with all the commitment and professionalism, which most probably earned you the promotion in the first place! Demonstrate your dedication to the practice by immersing yourself in your new position and show everyone how much you care about the business and how much you want it to thrive.

Naturally you can still remain friends as you did before but this new set of responsibilities means you now have to take control of certain aspects of their working life. In the past you could laugh and joke, be critical of others behind their backs, and even be derogatory (if you felt the need!) There now has to be an immediate cessation of this type of behaviour.

You have been identified by the owners as having the qualities necessary to lead and these past traits are not befitting of a leader. You have to set out the boundaries which your employees know you will not cross any longer. It's very difficult to be the joker and the friend, while still maintaining the gravitas and the dignity required to be an effective manager.

That said, this doesn't mean that you need to become isolated. You can and indeed must still be friendly with those you always have been but there now has to be a reduction in the number of occasions on which you act the fool. These boundaries are in place to enable you to create the environment which is essential for you to earn respect; and from this respect will soon come an acceptance that your role has changed.

Along with the larking around, so the gossip needs to be stopped too. Do not engage in idle chit chat about staff or the owners, as this is not conduct which befits a respected manager. The position of PM is one which needs to rise above this level of behind the back storytelling. Don't be concerned that your former colleagues notice this obvious change in your behaviour, as it all forms part of the process of your elevation from peer to authoritative leader.

One of the delegates on our recent year-long PM club programme is an established PM in Ireland and she has been through this exact process. Her tale is sure to resonate with a number of you:

The Dental Practice "Jugglers"

"I started as a trainee nurse, worked my way up, got the training, took on the head nurse position and then after a few years, the PM left and I was asked by the principal to interview for the position. I did have a background in business and marketing before I got into dentistry.

It was a challenge to move up from being a peer to a manager and even a few years on I'm still fighting that, even now every day, because there is still some of the original staff. I suppose it took a lot of time and a big change in mind-set and attitude.

You do have to make the decision and say, these people used to be my mates and we used to go out drinking but I'm not at that level with them anymore. You do have to take a step back and say – 'look guys, I know you don't like this but I do have to manage you, I'm being paid to manage you and although you don't like it, we need to find a way through this.'

People I would have been really good mates with and chatting to outside of work all the time, I don't socialise with at all.

I am comfortable with it because it's what I'm being paid to do. It was my choice to take on this role and I knew it was going to have an effect. You can't be best mates and surf the internet upstairs when nobody is looking; you have to change to be in this role, whether you like this or not."

As part of the elevation process, you should be noticeably more interested in *all* staff members and not simply those to whom who you were previously close. You need to ask everyone how they are doing, how they are feeling and engage them in conversation. It is important you start the process of relationship building

with those you have previously not truly befriended. You do not want to be accused of favouritism and this is one of the most effective ways of dispelling this perception.

The early stages of your new PM role is all about fact finding; not just about the job and what it entails but equally how the staff are coping with any changes which have occurred since you were promoted. It's vital to discover what other people think about this transitional stage, as you begin to establish your unique way of doing things.

As you begin your new role, why not prove you've listened to what staff members have been saying, by acting upon some of the issues they've described. You can't solve everything, but by picking your battles carefully, you can quickly be seen as someone who actually responds to improve situations that are affecting the morale of the practice.

While it is true that the role of PM should carry with it a certain degree of respect from those over whom you are now presiding, you still have to accept that there will be some of your colleagues who need time to be won over. Patience is the key here. Don't start to over analyse why some staff members don't seem to respect you while others do. It's important to understand in circumstances like this, that there will always be some who may not be happy with your promotion. Invariably, people don't like change and the practice has just seen a significant one, at managerial level.

It's possible at this very early stage, that there may be some who feel that the job has gone to the wrong person. Others may believe that they themselves have better credentials, or that one of their friends would have been better suited. You just have to accept that these opinions exist, sometimes purely out of jealousy.

The key factor to concentrate on as you seek to establish yourself as PM, is that the owners chose you; you certainly didn't assume the role or promote yourself to it. This factor alone should give you the self-confidence to proceed successfully, without the need for complete acceptance across the practice. There's a reason you were chosen by the owners and in the fullness of time you will prove that their choice was the wise one.

During this gradual process of gaining respect, it is imperative that you carry out your role without wavering. If you feel something needs to be changed, alter it. If you feel something needs to be said, say it! If you feel someone has stepped out of line, let them know that you won't tolerate it. All these things collectively will demonstrate that you have leadership qualities and that through these demonstrations of authority, you will begin the process of commanding the respect you deserve.

Through discussion, listening, coaching, mentoring, advising, improving and taking decisive action, will come a feeling of empathy, which will begin to endear you to even the most divisive colleague. You just have to accept that this may take a little longer with some colleagues, than it will with others. Stick to your excellent principles, exhibit your vast array of management skills and get on with being a great practice manager!

GENERAL RULES FOR NEWLY APPOINTED PMs

Whatever route you took to become the new PM, there are several basic principles which you may find useful as you seek to make your new position a great success.

A wonderful starting principle to bear in mind is that good management starts with good planning. Newly appointed PMs should have their goals and targets set for them, so make sure you have meaningful dialogue with the practice owner about what they are expecting from you. Try to pin them down to specifics wherever possible. It is much easier to make plans, when you are clear in your mind about what you are planning for.

New PMs should discuss with the owners what their vision is for the practice. What, for them are their aims and ambitions and how they would describe perfection. This will help you understand how the owners see their business and whether they have a realistic image of it.

You will only succeed if you and the owners have this shared vision. Your relationship with them will ultimately hold the key to your success. Be honest with them. Tell them what you expect from them and that you expect them to be there for you when required.

Ask them to present their long term goals and aspirations, so that you can establish the bigger picture beyond the day to day running of the practice. And don't make this the end of the dialogue; once these ideas have been formalised, arrange follow up meetings, scheduled or unscheduled, to ensure that they are pleased with your progress.

The Dental Practice "Jugglers"

While you are having these important discussions about the vision of the practice, it is also imperative that your role is carefully defined by your owner. You need to know where your responsibilities begin and end. It is as important to establish what areas you shouldn't become involved, as it is where you should. Let an owner explain what they believe comes under your remit and equally what doesn't.

One of the hardest things that a new PM will have to do is to begin to assert their authority. You need to be a balanced leader, as it is easy to come across as too autocratic on the one hand, or as a pushover on the other. By having these honest conversations with your owners it can help you to understand how best to achieve this. It's important for a new manager to establish with practice owners when they will step in and that you can call upon them when challenged.

Regardless of the ambitions of the owner, a new PM should always set themselves their own target of finding ways to improve productivity among the staff and reduce errors. You should attempt to develop staff skills and improve attitudes where necessary; you should also let staff know of your expectations.

As you set them their goals, you need to give employees a realistic amount of time to achieve them. You will ultimately need these targets to be reached and the more detail you can give them about the objective, the better equipped they'll be to realise it. Describe to employees a specific vision of what you want and then follow up with them when appropriate to see how they are progressing.

In time you should also be prepared to add new responsibilities to their roles if you can see they are capable and similarly be prepared to take responsibilities away if they aren't. You want them to succeed, so introduce new responsibilities slowly and steadily rather than swamp them. Gauge their progress and have follow up conversations, so they can describe how they are feeling about these new duties.

Despite these lofty, ambitious and idealistic aims and regardless of these significant initial conversations, it is still important to be realistic about the time scale involved. These are long term objectives and in some cases could take years not days.

Rest assured that not even the most driven business owner would expect you to be up to speed straight away and that they fully understand it's not realistic to have everything running smoothly from the outset. While you should expect to have a swift grasp of many things within your remit, a period of assessment is a minimum requirement, as you begin to establish exactly what it is that you are inheriting.

HOW TO GET THE MOST OUT OF THIS BOOK

Over the years we've worked with hundreds of different practices and have spent a great deal of time observing the many quirks and anomalies which differentiate one from another. Each business has its own unique challenges and its very specific needs. It would be churlish therefore to assemble a guidebook like this and expect it to solve all your varied issues.

That said, we are extremely confident that it provides a host of new ideas and creative solutions to the many shared difficulties which every business appears to face. You will read not just our thoughts and ideas but those of practice managers themselves and together we will guide you through the many aspects of this varied role.

With more than 30 years' experience between us of working within the dental profession we believe we are uniquely positioned to offer a genuine insight into this challenging industry and how best to maximise all it has to offer. In addition to the hundreds of hours we've spent working with dental professionals, we've conducted detailed research, speaking to dozens of industry professionals from right across the spectrum, in order to ensure that the contents of the book will resonate with every PM, no matter how much experience they've accumulated.

We believe that in order to have the greatest affect, it shouldn't simply be read once but should be readily accessible and referred to regularly as issues come and go within the practice. Our inspiration for writing this was born from the enormous admiration we have for the many talented PMs we've had the privilege of dealing with and how great is their desire to make their practice a success. In their insatiable quest to achieve all their goals, they've bombarded us with a range of pertinent questions and here within the pages of this book we have done our very best to answer them all. Enjoy!

Chapter 2

Presenting Change and Effective Communication

We've established in the opening chapter how your journey to the role of PM came about and the initial challenges which this complex role presents. What is clear is that whichever route you took to reach the position, you now fully understand how vital it is to make decisions and instigate change; now you need to be confident about the way in which you present those changes to your team.

There is an expectation that managers are idea originators. Often, a moment of inspiration will suddenly develop in their minds and before long a skilled PM can turn that random thought into a genuine proposition to improve the workings of the practice. As observers and overseers, nobody else possesses their unrivalled insight and it is through these observations that areas for improvement or enhancement can formulate. The next challenge of course is to articulate these ideas to those who need to implement it.

Managers are usually selected as a consequence of their array of diverse talents. Organisational and administrative qualities are a must, their determination and enthusiasm a pre-requisite. Many though, feel that the one area which can let them down is their ability to communicate, particularly in front of others.

There is little doubt that we are in an era where a lack of face to face communication is almost encouraged. The prevalence of texts and emails has created an environment in which relationships can be maintained without actually conversing with anybody. In a workplace, however, face to face communication is critical to the efficient running of a business.

Over the years, we've come across a worrying number of managers across many industries, whose reliance upon impersonal communiqués has ultimately led to their downfall. While the occasional memorandum is acceptable, using an email to consistently replace a face to face meeting quickly creates an unhealthy working atmosphere. Employees don't just need to hear from their managers, they want to see them too, if a genuine bond of trust is to be formed; and without this bond, the chances of a long term working relationship are negligible.

So why is it that some managers become faceless leaders, preferring to sit behind a closed office door and pump out an endless supply of emails, rather than engage with their staff? In the vast majority of cases, it all stems from a fundamental lack of confidence in their ability to communicate.

One of the great misconceptions is that the art of communication is entirely based on your genes; that somehow life determines whether you are born with the so-called "gift of the gab" and that those who feel they haven't been blessed in this way, are somehow condemned to being bashful and nervous talkers.

This simply isn't the case. Like most things in life, communication is a skill which can be acquired and improved; given the right coaching, allied to a determination to want to better themselves, almost anyone can improve their communication skills.

We are sometimes challenged about this bold statement and our advice is to give them a two hour homework assignment, insisting they watch the 2010 movie "The King's Speech". The film depicts the travails of King George VI, whose significant speech impediment is overcome thanks to the skilful work of an Australian speech therapist. (SPOILER ALERT! The emotional conclusion of this inspiring film is the brilliant speech delivered at the end, by a man who had previously thought such an oration was beyond him.)

This example is an extreme one of course and in the majority of cases the hurdles which have to be negotiated are far less complicated than a stammer. For most people, the most significant issue they face regarding their communication struggles, are actually psychological, as the mere prospect of speaking in front of others, fills them with dread.

It is widely accepted that one of the most common phobias which exists is the fear of public speaking. It is a genuine condition and has its own name *"glossophobia"*. There's even been a claim that as many as 75% of adults have this condition – more than fear death! American comedian Jerry Seinfeld once joked, that more people in attendance at a funeral would prefer to be in the coffin, than deliver the eulogy!

The Dental Practice "Jugglers"

When you delve into the reasons why this genuine fear exists, sufferers point to a series of irrational expectations that they will dry up or be ridiculed; for others it is the mere thought of being the centre of attention which is sufficient to transform them into a nervous wreck.

The expectations on a PM are certainly not as dramatic as a stammering King broadcasting to the nation ahead of the Second World War but there is little doubt that the prospect for some of delivering certain edicts to their staff, still carries with it a degree of anxiety. Many PMs actually find this aspect of their job the most challenging and we have come across many who have sleepless nights ahead of most team meetings; almost without expectation that fear of falling flat is at the root of their restlessness.

One of the first steps to being able to dismiss these baseless fears is an understanding of why PMs are in the position of having to issue the edicts in the first place. If we go back to the original paragraph of this chapter, we described managers as idea generators and talked about how their unique position, allowed them to gauge where change was necessary, to improve the efficiency of the practice.

If the idea being delivered, therefore, is a PMs, then who better to describe it than the PM themselves? Nobody has better insight, nobody can explain the thought process that was behind it more succinctly and there's nobody else with a greater knowledge of why it's going to benefit the practice; you are, after all, the person who identified why the idea was necessary in the first place. It is clear therefore, that you *are* the best person for this presentation task.

Despite knowing this to be true, there are still many PMs who view the whole communication process itself as a chore which has to be done, rather than an opportunity to exhibit their leadership qualities. It can often be born from an inaccurate and overly critical view of those who are about to be in their audience – in other words, their staff.

For many PMs, the lack of self-belief in their own communication skills, actually stems from a mistakenly held belief that they aren't respected enough by their subordinates. In these circumstances it can be beneficial ahead of any team meeting, to take a moment to think again about why you are in the position of manager at your practice.

As we've already pointed out, (and are delighted to do so again!), almost without exception, a PM is in their role because someone has appointed them; at some point, when seeking to fill this pivotal role within their business, an owner has identified your qualities ahead of any other. They believe that you are the ideally suited individual to look after their precious practice. They identified, among many other qualities within you, this amazing gift of being able to generate ideas to improve their business - now is the opportunity to describe and implement one such idea to your staff.

This factor alone should carry with it a sense of pride and with it a realisation that it commands inherent respect within the practice. Staff should view you as their leader and what better way of a leader demonstrating those leadership skills, than by the origination, delivery and ultimate implementation of an idea to improve the workings of a business?

If all that hasn't galvanised you, then there's another good reason why you should feel that your staff will view you with respect whenever you speak to them at a team meeting – that many of them would rather die than speak in front of other people! If 75% of adults have a public speaking phobia, the chances are that most of those gathered, wouldn't dream of being the centre of attention in front of their colleagues. The mere fact that you have the guts to stand up and impart instruction and information to them, demonstrates a quality that marks you out as the head of the team.

We accept that communication is an extremely broad topic. We have naturally only been able to skim the surface of the range of psychological issues which can hamper successful presentation. Perhaps though, you will still be able to identify with some of those we have highlighted; now the next step to improving your communication is to look at the practical side of successful presentation.

Something which is often overlooked by managers before they embark on any presentation, is the significance of planning and preparation. As individuals, managers are notoriously meticulous in their procedures when it comes to any aspect of their working life, yet they don't seem to embark on those same levels of preparation when it comes to articulating new ideas to their team. This situation has to be reversed. Benjamin Franklin once famously said, "By failing to prepare, you are preparing to fail." It's an adage which is well known to successful people across every walk of life.

As regular public speakers and presenters ourselves, we have a series of important stages which we embark upon before we reach the point at which we feel ready to present; and these stages apply whether we are talking for two minutes or two hours, to two people or to two thousand!

The first thing we do is to regularly revisit our

presentations and ultimately this leads to a series of re-writes, as we seek to improve our words. We are effectively editing our work, looking for better words and phrases, and checking that what we've written makes sense, while equally finding ways to make it more concise. One of the golden rules is to try and use fewer words wherever possible, as to be more concise, has a powerful impact on any presentation.

It is widely accepted that people generally have short attention spans and that their ability to digest and process information is limited. We therefore have to be precise with the details of the communication we are conveying. We need to be as succinct as possible and make sure that what we say has the impact we require.

When a PM delivers a new idea, it is even more imperative that they apply these principles, as ultimately their aim is for the staff to perform a task differently to how they were doing it before. The fewer pieces of information they have to digest, the easier it will be for them to understand what they have to do. The more concise the communiqué, the likelier it will be that they can carry out this new way of working.

We often say that an excellent way of judging whether a PM has delivered an edict well, is by the number of questions they are asked about it afterwards. If there are a host of questions about seemingly simple elements of this new working practice, the chances are you've failed to communicate it successfully. If, however, questions are few and when you are asked you can reply with the phrase, *"As I said in my presentation…."* you know that the issue is with their listening skills and *not* with your communication.

Another part of the preparation procedure is to practice the actual delivery of your presentation. Whether it be in front of a mirror or in front of a trusted friend or family member, rehearsal is essential. No manager should ever be in a situation where the first time they present a communication is when they do it for real.

You need to know that it reads well, sounds right, and that you are comfortable with your choice of phraseology. In truth there is no other way of finding that out, than by delivering what you've written. No matter the length of the material, you have to become so familiar with it, that you know it practically off by heart. In truth, some of the best presenters we've ever come across have been able to do exactly that – present without anything written down!

It is also vital to become aware of the best stance to adopt when you are delivering. Most people know of the significance of body language and eye contact when it comes to communication with others, yet they neglect its importance when it comes to presentation delivery. Keeping an open stance, with your head raised is one of the keys to effective communication and will maximise the opportunity for eye contact with your staff. If you want your employees to absorb what you're telling them, you need to look at them as often as possible, hence the reason why presenters without scripts have such a powerful effect on their audience.

We do accept that for many PMs, the presence of a script of some sort is a must but the key to the script you have at your fingertips is how easy it is to glance at, in order to maintain maximum eye contact. A script can become a "crutch" rather than a necessity for the well-rehearsed presenter, so if you feel you simply can't deliver without one, make sure it is as succinct as possible.

We always recommend a "bullet point" script rather

than a fully worded manuscript; so rather than full sentences written down on several pieces of paper, try putting short prompts together on one piece of paper. This will act as a guide to your presentation, rather than a verbose blow by blow account of the idea you are introducing to the practice and will allow you to lift your head with regularity. Remember that these ideas are your own, so brief prompts should be all you need to remind you of the points you are making.

In our experience, one of the most common reasons why presenters let themselves down during a presentation, is that they lose their place in a lengthily written script and can't find where they are up to; the sight of a panic-stricken presenter, frantically flicking through their copious notes, is usually the obvious indicator. A bullet point prompt will instantly eradicate this commonly occurring problem; and the key to being able to be this concise, is to ensure that your presentation has the right structure.

On our courses, when we are dealing with PMs on the issue of improved communication skills, they will commonly point to the number of times at which they've been guilty of waffle. They will describe a team meeting which began effectively, only to degenerate into an incomprehensible and largely confusing mass of confusing gibberish! It's negative experiences like this which can quickly convince a PM that they aren't good communicators, when in reality, it has come about for one very simple and easily rectifiable reason – they've not put a good enough structure to their presentation.

When it comes to delivering a presentation of whatever length, the success of its impact can often depend upon its structure. As a rule, a presentation without a defined structure is much more likely to lead to failure, with its presenter often losing the thread and ultimately reverting to a vague, disconnected period of unintelligible babble – in other words WAFFLE!

For many years, Alistair has been delivering a hugely successful confidence building course, aimed at tackling those for whom public speaking would be the source of nightmares – *"Breakthrough Day – Develop Self-Confidence"*. As the delegates begin their day long journey with him, they describe the reasons why the very notion of public speaking has become their nemesis. For many, it is that graphic image of themselves, hopelessly losing their way in mid-talk; and in every case where this is the source of their fears, they soon admit to being unaware of the significance of a well-defined structure.

You may never have thought about it but structured communication has been a part of our lives since we were babies. From the day we first nestle on our mother's lap as she reads us a bed time story, we quickly become familiar with the concept of structured storytelling. Every tale we hear, no matter how primitive, has a clear beginning, a carefully constructed middle and an unmistakeable ending.

At the beginning we hear a *"Once Upon A Time…"* which lets us know that the story has begun; in the middle we hear descriptions of the characters, the emotions they are feeling and the drama of the tale as it unfolds; and at the end we await the moment when we know that fairy tale has concluded, *"…and they all lived, happily ever after."* These same principles of structure have to be applied in every piece of communication we ever deliver.

While naturally a PM won't be beginning their communiqué with a *"Once Upon A Time…"* it is vital that they think carefully of a strong opening which lets the staff know that they need to pay attention to what's being said. It needs to be both powerful and clear, as the impact, has to grab their attention from the outset. We often advise our PMs to cut out the *"thanks for coming…"* and the *"I appreciate you getting here early…"* in favour of an immediate attention-grabbing *"As of Tuesday 3rd June we will be……"*. Starting in this no-nonsense way will quickly establish your presence and ensure that all phones are put down and chatting will cease.

The middle section of any presentation contains all the detail of the new working practice you are introducing. Although that has to be informative, it also needs to be precise. We described earlier that people's attention spans are minimal, so it is imperative that a strict editing process has been undertaken, with every effort made to be concise and punchy. If you need to include facts and figures, make them brief and easily digestible. Be mindful that your staff will be hearing your new idea for the first time, so the less the detail they have to absorb, the greater understanding they will have of what you are proposing.

To ensure the perfect conclusion to your presentation, you need to make sure that your ending has these four vital components.

1) It is a brief summary of what has preceded it.
2) It is similar to your opening.
3) It is succinct.
4) It is definitive.

If you think of your ending as being the final thing your audience will hear, it needs to be memorable; and for it to be memorable, it needs to have been carefully constructed. It is such a vital part of the process, that on his presentation and public speaking courses, Alistair always encourages delegates to begin writing their endings before any other part of their presentation. A good ending will both enhance the presentation and drive home the message you set out to impart. Ensure, therefore, that you give it the attention it merits.

But what if, after all this excellent work has been carried out perfectly, that your staff still won't buy into your new concept? What if, despite adhering to all the correct principles and utilising the structure efficiently, that there is still cynicism among your team?

You may have come to work that day full of enthusiasm and excitement, ready to share a new idea, only to end it feeling deflated and maybe even angry.

Well here's a four-step approach that can help you deal with these objections and will begin to turn even the most negative team member around.

The most important thing to remember first and foremost is not to adopt a defensive stance. It is imperative that you keep calm and maintain a dignified exterior. The great diffuser in these situations is to begin to demonstrate empathy and to try to see things from their point of view.

For the purpose of this exercise, let's use the example that you want to start answering the telephone at lunch times. Up to this point practice policy has always been to close for lunch but after years of having this break in the day, you are now looking to change this completely, by having the telephone answered at this time.

It is essential, therefore, that you demonstrate empathy with this significant change to their routine as quickly as possible. And you can do this by saying:

"I understand your concerns, as being concerned about it is perfectly understandable and normal."

By communicating this type of language, it shows that you have listened and that you understand their point of view. This will immediately instil a sense, that not only have they been listened to, but that you accept their right to be concerned about this major upheaval.

The second step is to ask questions and gather more information about their concern. It is often the case that our interpretation of their feelings can be inaccurate or that they may have not actually meant what they have said. In order to move forward we need to establish exactly why they are objecting and not simply make assumptions.

You can do this by asking a simple question such as: *"Tell me why you feel it won't work?"* Or, *"tell me why you feel this way?"* It is then essential that you listen attentively to their answer, as you need to fully understand their concerns.

They may respond by saying that it will remove the opportunity to bond and socialize, or perhaps that the phone is relatively quiet during lunchtimes anyway. At this point, the key is to summarize back to them what they have told you. *"So you are concerned that it may have an impact on your bonding and socializing?"* Once they confirm this is their objection, you are then ready to move to stage three, in the knowledge that you know the real reason for their concern.

It is now time to answer that concern but in order to do so you must have already done all the necessary homework in advance, so that you have the required facts at your disposal to overcome their resistance.

We recently received a call from a client with this very issue, who had the idea for a lunchtime rota after attending our Reception Programme, *"How to turn enquiries into appointments."*

She had received some resistance from her team in the past to this concept but she was determined to try to introduce it. We advised her to call a meeting with her team to discuss the issue but ahead of doing so, to have done at least one of these two things beforehand:

Either

1. Answer the phone herself for a period of time in order to measure how many calls the practice typically receives during lunchtime.
   AND/OR
2. To leave the answer machine on and see how many people called during that time and then actually left a message when they did. (In our experience the percentage of people who actually leave messages is negligible).

   She opted to answer the telephone herself for two weeks and she then shared the results with the team. During that period, she managed to convert 11 new enquires into appointments. It was at a rate of better than one a day. We often say that each new patient is worth at least £3000 to a practice if they stay with you for ten years, so simply by answering calls herself during lunchtime she may have earned her practice £33,000! These kinds of facts and figures formed the basis of a very solid argument as to why she was introducing this new lunchtime answering policy.

(She even went a step further and has employed a telephone answering company to answer their calls for them outside work hours; it meant that effectively they are now a 24 hours a day practice. It has already made a significant impact on the number of new patients visiting the practice, as so many people do their internet surfing in evenings and at weekends.)

In order therefore, to ensure that you get a positive reaction from your team you need to gather as much data as possible. Change is usually a source of great concern to employees whose natural reaction is to be uncomfortable and ultimately negative towards it. Detailed facts and figures may not immediately make them like the change but will certainly make them realize exactly why they need to accept it.

Having discussed their concerns more empathetically and added greater detail as to why it is happening, the fourth step is to ask them what they now think about your idea, armed with this additional information. It is important at this point to try and gauge whether they have any ideas which may allow it to be introduced more smoothly. Ask for suggestions and perhaps even allow them to take some ownership of the new policy.

In the example we outlined earlier, the client told the team to come up with their own rota and within a day it had been arranged and implemented. In effect, by allowing the staff to take ownership of one aspect of this new change it will feel less of an imposition. We always advise in these circumstances to try and let the team have a say in handling the new concept. Employees are much more likely to embrace a change to their working life, when they feel that their own ideas have played a part in shaping it.

So here are the four steps to overcoming objections to change:

Step one - Show empathy.

Step two - Ask more questions about their concerns to fully understand them.

Step three- provide a solution with as much data and information as possible to back up your plan.

Step Four- gauge their reactions, ask for ideas and work together on moving forward.

As we've demonstrated throughout this chapter, improving communication skills in the workplace is a complex task. There is such a myriad of different aspects to it, that there are countless books that have been written solely on this subject alone.

What we have tried to do here, is to tailor it to suit the specific needs of a PM within their role at the practice. The tips and ideas we have shared are of necessity brief and concise. We strongly recommend that you seek further guidance by enrolling onto one of our communication courses, where you will receive bespoke one to one coaching with us. More details of which can be found in the appendix section of this book.

… with your communication skills honed, you should now

CHAPTER 3

Productive Meetings

With your communication skills honed, you should now be feeling empowered to embark on one of the key areas in which confident presentation is an essential asset and that is to conduct a team meeting.

Every PM should be aware of the importance of gathering their team together for regular staff meetings. Love them or loathe them, they are a vital tool in ensuring that everyone within the practice is aware of the goings on within the business.

In our experience, we've yet to encounter a practice which doesn't hold them, albeit the regularity with which they are held varies dramatically from business to business.

For example, one of the practices we deal with have a daily mini meeting or "team huddle" fifteen minutes before the day's first appointment; they have a more formal weekly, hour long meeting every Friday, when the practice is closed, to allow a full catch up of the week's events and a throw forward to the following week; and a monthly meeting on the final Wednesday of each month to look at longer term strategies – this too occurs with the practice closed for its duration.

Contrast that with a practice we encountered recently in which meetings were held, at most, once a month on an ad hoc basis, with the real possibility of it being cancelled altogether if the practice was busy.

We are often asked by PMs what the ideal number of meetings should be and without wishing to sit on the fence, our answer is that it depends on the effectiveness of the communication methods of the business. In other words, a meeting is a method of articulating information to your staff and if the existing lines of communication are frequent and clear, this will affect the number of formal meetings which are necessary.

That said, you should never underestimate the psychological effect of regular meetings either, as these get-togethers are vital to promote a sense of collective bonding within the team. Team huddles are a powerful force in promoting morale.

So, having established the importance of meetings, it is now essential that these gatherings are as effective and productive as possible.

Ask yourself if you have ever sat in a meeting where you wished you hadn't turned up? Or worse still, that you've held a meeting which has completely bombed!

As PM, have you walked into a room full of enthusiasm, seeking inspiration and ideas from your team, only to be left bewildered and deflated by the end?

Let's take a look at these scenarios to see if they sound familiar:

- Many ideas were discussed at the meeting; however weeks and months later none of the ideas were then implemented.
- A meeting that was supposed to last an hour overran dramatically, yet most of the team didn't say anything at all.
- You sat in a meeting and started to wonder if an email would have sufficed.
- You concluded that staff were reluctant to share new ideas.
- Only one or two senior team members seemed to be dominating the conversation.
- It ended up becoming little more than a bitching and moaning session, with very few useful issues concluded.

If this has happened to you, don't despair as there is a great deal that can be done to rectify it; instead of giving up, concentrate on why it's so important to turn all these negatives around:

1. The bonding element. People are usually so busy in the practice, that many don't get a chance to sit down and discuss ideas together.
2. If you get good ideas from your team, they feel they have had an impact and can make a difference.
3. They feel valued because their opinions count.
4. Your team are more likely to run with new ideas if they were theirs in the first place!
5. You can actually get some good solutions to some of the challenges you face – remember you don't hold the exclusivity on all problem solving!

6. It is a good way of improving the patient journey within the practice. If people get on well together, then it will improve the patient journey.

Like anything within business, creating productive meetings are something which can be worked on, provided you are determined to try something different.

Here are list of ideas which can transform your practice get-togethers:

1) Set an agenda

Your agenda will set expectations, chart a clear direction and give people a chance to prepare for your meeting. Share it at least a few days in advance.

Don't just list the topics you want to cover: instead, make a note of things on which you'd like others to provide input.

Giving people an agenda beforehand gives them time to think about ideas, so they aren't coming into it cold.

2) Time

Be strict on time, so if the meeting is from 8 – 9, then make sure it sticks to these parameters.

Ensuring you keep to the correct timing is crucial, as once you go over, people's minds usually start to wander; this is particularly the case if it is a Friday afternoon meeting – nobody wants time eaten away from their weekends.

In our experience running a meeting on a Friday afternoon is never a good idea, as by then, staff will invariably already be thinking about the weekend and will be much less inclined to want to extend the meeting with their ideas!

3) **Ground Rules**

It is your meeting, so you are entitled to set some ground rules. Here are a few which we encourage:
- No mobiles- say no more!
- Ensure that everyone is on time. Start the meeting on time even if there are only half the people in the room; this will embarrass anyone that is late.
- No food- it's an unnecessary and sometimes noisy distraction!
- Make sure you provide paper and pens. This is important for note taking and will prevent those who would otherwise make notes on their smart phones.
- Invest in a flip chart; this is imperative as you write ideas down from your team. (You will shortly find out why this will be a very worthwhile investment.)

One of the keys to promoting a productive and ultimately successful meeting is by garnering ideas from your team; and by team, we mean everyone, not just the confident members!

Too often when we have observed PMs holding a meeting, they seek out ideas, only to be met with a stony, uncomfortable silence. Even issues as significant as how to improve patient numbers, fail to provoke a response; or if it does, it is from the same person who always contributes at team meetings, while others sit with their mouths tightly closed.

Here's a formula to overcome this, which we've used for many years and which has produced some stunning results:

The first thing you need to do is to split the team into smaller groups.

Let's say for example you have 12 team members - put them into three teams of four; then appoint a leader for each team and ideally select the quietest person for the role; (the rationale behind this, is that it is really helpful in developing their own personal growth.)

At this point you need to ask the relevant questions once again and to set each team the task of originating their ideas to the team leader in five minutes: every member of the group has to come up with at least one idea.

The major advantage of following this process is that you will promote a number of fresh ideas from the shyer members of the team, who feel much more confident about contributing in the smaller size group.

The ultimate purpose of this exercise is simply to get as many ideas as possible; therefore at this stage ensure that the group doesn't discuss them in detail but merely collates them with a brief explanatory outline.

If you've explained yourself effectively, you will then witness three groups enthusiastically chatting away; perhaps set a challenge to see which group originates the most ideas.

Once the five minutes is up, ask each team leader to stand up at their place and share their ideas. At this point it is imperative that you don't exhaust one team leader's ideas, as you will then struggle to get more from the other two groups. Simply request five ideas from the first team leader, five from the next and so on until all the ideas have been discussed; this is certain to lead to a flip chart full of ideas.

Initially as you write them up, it is important not to discuss them, as at this point all you want is a number of original thoughts; don't say, *"that's a good idea"* or *"I'm not sure that will work"*, as you want to create a positive environment, so that team members will see the value in making contributions in the future.

When all the ideas have been written down, complement the teams on their productivity and give out positive feedback, especially to the team leaders for their role in the exercise.

Only once all the ideas have been written down is it time to discuss them in detail and when you do, make sure that you are as positive as possible throughout.

For example, if you feel you have to dismiss an idea because it will exceed your budget, then explain that while it is a good thought, you don't currently have the money to pursue it – perhaps state that you will make a note of it, to implement if things change in the future.

At the conclusion of the meeting, the next thing you must do is to actually attempt to implement these ideas; or at the very least to carry out some follow up action. If you want the team to feel as though they haven't wasted their time, they need to see their efforts have been acted upon.

In truth, if you attempt to run with one of the ideas that originated from the team meeting, then you will see a much greater level of enthusiasm from them as they'll effectively be pursuing one of their own creative thoughts! As with anything else though, keep an eye on its progress and be sure to arrange a follow up meeting to monitor its success.

By following these steps, we can promise you a much more positive outcome to your team meetings, with both a greater sense of total participation and a list of encouraging fresh ideas.

One of the PMs on our recent year-long PM club programme tried this technique to pep up her team meetings and was blown away by the response:

"I ran a meeting with the team on how to grow patient numbers. I decided to do something different and hold it outside as it was such a warm day. There were six of us in that day, so I split the teams into two groups of three and put the question of patient numbers to them in greater detail.

The two groups were then tasked with creating as many ideas as possible and were given ten minutes to discuss it. Once they finished, I got all the ideas down from the two groups and as a result they'd actually come up with 18 new ideas; they ranged from handing out referral cards to doing a wedding shower!

It was definitely one of the most productive meetings I have ever run."

The Morning Huddle

Probably one of the most important types of team meeting you can facilitate is the morning huddle; this is where you have an opportunity to gather the team together and discuss the day's forthcoming events. We are surprised at how many practices don't take part in this vital bonding ritual, the advantages of which are numerous.

The main purpose of this excellent exercise is to discuss the patients who have appointments that day; this offers a chance not only to discuss how best to treat them but can additionally allow the team to open their minds to any potential marketing strategies for the practice (we will describe this in more detail shortly.)

On our "*Reception Course*" one day programme, we coach the front desk team on how to turn an enquiry into an appointment. We reveal a more rigid, structured approach and our clients have reported remarkable successes using these strategies.

During the day, each delegate must complete a *"telephone answering sheet"*, which asks a number of questions, requiring at least six pieces of information to be gathered about each patient who calls in. We then challenge the receptionist who takes these details, to give a small verbal presentation at a morning huddle, so that the entire team can be fully informed about the patient in question. To complete the task, they must then hand over the information sheet to either the TCO, PM or the dentist accordingly.

By completing this cycle of events it will mean that it won't just be the receptionist who will know the wants and needs of each patient but the entire team; this excellent discipline then allows a genuine rapport to be built up by whichever staff member greets the patient when they arrive and ensures that the practice can create an excellent first impression.

Over the years practices have told us of the incredible impact this simple procedure has had on their patients. Imagine how they feel when their dentist asks them about a forthcoming wedding, or how a new job is going, when they first enter a surgery. This kind of genuine interest engenders a real sense of care about each individual, well beyond their oral health alone.

The additional bonus is that the receptionist who started the whole information gathering process, will also feel that they've played a significant part in creating this rapport and will have a greater understanding of how key their role is to the practice and the impact they can have. It's why we refer to them as the *"managing directors of first impressions"* whenever they attend our reception course.

Another must at the morning huddle is to discuss patients who are set to complete their treatment, or are about to have a follow-up appointment. These two scenarios offer an excellent opportunity to request video testimonials and letters. When patients successfully complete their treatment they are most likely to be at their happiest and will be at their most receptive to the idea of a testimonial. This concept of reciprocation is a well-accepted and indeed proven concept within business. There is a widely held view that when asking for a favour at this point, patients will have a sense of obligation to agree to your request; the same applies equally to handing out referral cards too.

As well as offering an ideal platform to discuss patients' special needs or requirements, the morning huddle is also when tasks can be delegated and issues can be raised. It should be a largely informal occasion, the boundaries for which should always be flexible to accommodate any matters of concern. Though your time will naturally be limited as the day's first appointments loom, these topics for discussion can ultimately form the agenda of a more formal meeting at a later date and will give the team a real sense that there is a genuine forum for all their concerns.

In truth these huddles have become little short of a significant team bonding session; they can be uplifting and if held properly can create a genuine sense of togetherness and collective responsibility. (On one of Ashley's recent visits to the USA, he even witnessed one practice sing a practice song to round off the session!)

In our experience, practices who make the morning huddle part of the fabric of their regular routine, generally are the ones who have the highest morale and the most contented staff. If it's not already part of your daily routine, then it should be!

Chapter 4

Staff Motivation

It won't come as a surprise to any manager to learn that staff who are motivated, are statistically proven to perform better than those who are not. The most important factor to consider though is that what represents motivation for one person, may offer little motivation for another. It's absolutely pivotal therefore, for a PM to get to know their staff members, in order to determine what makes them tick.

Many PMs believe that motivation is purely based on monetary reward, but while naturally most employees will be at work in order to provide for their families, it's by no means their sole motivational force.

For some people, it could be a sense of belonging and being valued, for others it may be an opportunity to better themselves as individuals; in a field like dentistry it could be that some are there hoping to selflessly offer care to others. It's one of the key challenges for any PM, to try to understand each employee's "raison d'être".

In any working environment, it is vital that an employee

first and foremost, feels valued. If an individual doesn't feel their role within the practice has any significance, it is sure to have a negative effect on their motivation.

The first way a PM can make an employee feel that value, is by letting them know that you've noticed what they've done. Praise is always a great starting point, albeit they must deserve it. To simply complete a task, in itself, isn't usually enough to earn a compliment but if the manner in which it has been done has impressed you, then let them know. Too often a PM will be quick to point out an employee's error but rarely be as swift to acknowledge when they've excelled; staff that are praised for their contributions, are sure to be more motivated.

Another way of making a staff member know they are valued is by ensuring they have the tools necessary for them to do their job efficiently. Too often an employee is presented with a task that should be within their compass, only to be hampered by a lack of resources, a lack of support from you, or maybe a lack of time. An employee who has both the right equipment and the right support, will again feel motivated. In some cases, support should extend to include the right training. If a staff member tells you that they feel they would benefit from formal training, you should certainly do what you can to organise it for them.

Financial rewards can of course be a major driving force in motivating staff, but again, to simply think in terms of a pay increase is far too simplistic. In truth, those who only think in this way, are unlikely to succeed in truly raising morale. PMs need to think much more creatively when it comes to bonuses and rewards, as more money often has only a fleeting boost to an employee's motivation. For the sceptics among you, (and I'm sure there will be many), it's important to think about a pay rise, not in a psychological way but purely in a mathematical way.

Let's say for example that you have a staff member on a salary of £18,000 who has mentioned in a number of previous appraisals that they believe they would be a lot happier if they had a pay rise. In order to raise their morale, you eventually decide to award them a very generous 10% pay rise taking them up to £19800. In simple terms it means that before tax they will be earning an extra £150 a month. After tax, it means their take home pay will increase by £25 a week. In terms of long term motivation this is surely unlikely to have the desired morale boosting effect you are hoping for.

While pay increases are a must in order to at least keep pace with inflation and the rising cost of living, PMs need to think much more deeply about its motivational effect. After all, if you are generous enough to offer a pay increase as large as 10%, the likelihood is that there won't be another pay increase for some time after.

As a general principle in our experience, pay rewards can work as a motivational tool with staff who are already diligent, as it helps them strive to be even better; by contrast it will rarely work on an employee who is simply going through the motions.

A PM on a recent year- long programme with us, not only agreed with that principle but also believes that the way in which a pay increase is introduced, can inspire hard working employees to excel still further:

"We don't have employee of the month but the owner is

very generous with regular pay rises and bonuses. It is a well-known fact within the practice that if you work hard, are over performing and giving more than just what is expected, then you will get a pay rise. You could even get a pay rise every other month here and there's also the possibility of a one off bonus as well.

There is no fast and fixed rule regarding those bonuses. We just say that a person has done really well, let's give them a bonus; and you see how much it motivates because they don't know when it's going to happen.

You call them in and say, listen we really appreciate what you have done and there's a little bit extra in your pay cheque this month.

Because they didn't expect it, it means so much more to them; they've been recognised, without it being at a certain time of the year – like 31st December or whatever.

Pay rises don't though work with unmotivated staff. A pay rise will NEVER solve any motivational problem. If they aren't motivated to work, it will not do anything. We have actually had staff say to us – listen I don't care, you can give me all the money in the world but that will not change my attitude to this place."

As mentioned earlier, therefore, you need to give greater thought to what rewards will have a longer lasting effect on your staff. One excellent way in which you can reward staff who go that extra mile, is with extra days off, or additional days of annual leave. It's up to you how you decide what staff need to do in order to attain these bonus days but as long as an employee can see a tangible method of achieving it, it is sure to have a motivational effect.

You could perhaps link extra days off to an "employee

of the month" system in which a series of criteria, such as positive feedback from colleagues and patients, leads to the monthly accolade. While initially the winning employee should receive a less extravagant reward, such as a spa day or a meal out, accumulatively over a 12 month period, a series of employee of the month awards will then ultimately lead to the bigger prize of extra days off.

With this longer term goal at the "finish line" it can maintain motivation for a sustained period of time, than any "quick fix" pay rise. This longer term situation also allows a PM plenty of time in which to plan their rotas accordingly, to ensure that the winning employee's potential time off, isn't going to leave the practice stretched. Naturally the time off, when it comes, has to be at an agreed time with both parties.

There are some practices which don't have any financial or tangible rewards as a tool for motivation, preferring instead to build morale through social events and bonding days. A PM at one such practice we deal with, believes these days out have been working well:

"We always have a summer and a Christmas function; we do things like go-karting, as well as drinks and food, so it's a team exercise, where we can create some competitiveness, amidst the fun. We've done a day at the races; we celebrate birthdays and though these things seem small, they do go a long way towards making you feel as though you are a part of a team and that you can rely on each other.

Additionally we also celebrate success, so in terms of passing a cqc inspection for example, we may celebrate that, and say thanks for the daily work that they do.

These things will all help with motivation when you don't

have a bonus scheme. We will make most of these bonding days on work days too, so that we shut the practice and take them out on a normal working day. We will of course pay for everything on their behalf and make sure it costs them nothing."

Another motivational strategy can be to give a staff member more responsibilities. If handled in the right way, rather than being seeing as an extra burden, it can actually demonstrate your recognition that the he/she has exhibited such a high standard of work in their existing duties, that you feel they have the skills necessary to take on even greater challenges. The key to it, is the way in which this new area of responsibility is presented.

Let's take the case of a receptionist who has demonstrated wonderful people skills. Her empathy with the patients and willingness to go the extra mile on their behalf, has not only made her popular with them but means she has become a real boon for you.

Why not give the employee concerned an extra range of duties, which involve more interaction with your patients? Perhaps put her in charge of gathering and collating patient feedback sheets? Better still, bring her in on this project much earlier and allow her to make a contribution to devising these new patient feedback sheets during the planning stage.

Why not create a new extra title for her, such as the practice's first ever "patient journey co-ordinator"? If you do, make sure that this new title is awarded in a five minute coronation ceremony in front of all the staff, with a celebratory cake and a brief speech from the owner. While this may sound excessive, it actually sends out a very powerful message to all the staff, that those who put in the kind of effort that helps the practice excel, are not only recognised but rewarded for their efforts. This one extremely visible action alone, can help to motivate the entire practice, not just the individual, successful employee.

While this situation does not actually involve a genuine promotion, the prospect of moving up the ladder is always an area of motivation for ambitious employees, who can see that there is a genuine career path within the practice. Receptionists can become head receptionists, nurses can become lead nurses, lead nurses can become treatment co-ordinators and so on. It is important that all employees within the practice are aware of these career paths and equally that these promotions are not simply based on who is the oldest or has been there the longest.

A PMs motto has to be, "if you are good enough, you are old enough". Too often within practices, those who have been there the longest become the "head" of their respective area, when in actuality there are far better equipped employees, overlooked by virtue of their age or length of service. While it isn't easy for a PM to promote a younger, inexperienced employee ahead of one with longer service, it is essential that the criteria used to determine who is moved upwards, is based solely on their ability to do the job.

Many PMs, in a bid to avoid an uncomfortable conversation and fearful of the inevitable negative reaction of the overlooked staff member, prefer to play it safe and promote the senior member, even if they are acutely aware that a younger employee is far better equipped to excel in the position.

In reality, this can be a mistake as, short term pain, will ultimately become long term gain. A PM who hasn't promoted well, will merely be adding to their own workload, as the inevitable deficiencies of the promoted employee, will mean a much less efficient area of the practice. This will then necessitate the PMs regular intervention and in all likelihood lead to a series of confrontations with the employee concerned. In effect, by avoiding one potentially awkward conversation initially, the PM will actually have created a number of regular blow-outs further down the line.

A PM at one of the smaller practices we deal with is convinced that because there is only a small staff, what they want to see above everything else, is that the PM is seen to be "mucking in" with the rest of the team:

"In terms of motivating them, they are very much aware that we work as a team and I wouldn't expect them to do anything that I wouldn't do myself; I think that's important for them to know. I think some people in a managerial position feel that they've worked their way up the ladder and they don't now need to do the tasks that staff members can do; but I feel that it's a matter of working together to get the job done.

As well as that, I also ensure that I keep them aware of what's happening and what's relevant to the practice. There are obviously certain things they wouldn't be able to know but I think if they are aware of what's going on, are involved to a certain extent, they feel part of the team and are happy to do their utmost to ensure that we succeed.

It may be we have survived without a bonus scheme because we are quite small. I am very quick to advise the individual staff members if they are mentioned personally, in feedback we've received from a patient. I make sure that they're aware of all the feedback that has come in for us as a team and the fact that we do a great job for our patients. No monetary or physical rewards exist. There's no points system or prizes available- none of that."

It's clear that motivation can come in many forms; as with so many things in a working environment, no single business can claim to have the exclusive recipe. While a bonus scheme may work for some, regular minor incentives like days out may work for another; it very much depends on the personalities within your practice and the atmosphere they collectively create.

Whichever formula work best, make sure you don't offer these perks too readily or that they can be achieved too easily, as what once was something which staff aspired to, can quickly become something they expect; if they expect it, you can be sure it won't motivate them any longer and you will soon be back at square one!

CHAPTER 5

Coaching, Mentoring and Feedback

As a PM you should be aware of the significance of being a supportive coach to your employees, assisting, guiding and advising them where appropriate. Being a manager is as much about improving people, as it is managing them.

While coaching should be a naturally continuing process, the most widely accepted method of keeping track of staff development, is by utilising dedicated lines of communication through regular appraisals.

Appraisals (or 1-2-1s) should be conducted on at least a quarterly basis. They need to be a formal occasion, with a confirmed appointment, which staff should know about, at least two weeks in advance.

Give them a form to fill out ahead of each meeting with appropriate questions such as, *"What has gone well since we last we met? What hasn't? What would you like to achieve in the next quarter? Is there anything you'd like to change in the next quarter? Are there any areas of your job which we could help to improve?"*

These meetings should always be one to one (without an owner in the room) and behind closed doors. Once concluded, you should jot down the minutes and get the staff member to sign off on them, as being an accurate reflection of what has been said. These can ultimately be added to their personnel files and can be used as documented evidence of your employee's progress and conduct at the practice.

Appraisals should be used to evaluate each employee's performance. Their strengths should be identified, their weaknesses assessed and methods to improve them offered. Training should be discussed if necessary and there should be formal goals set by specific dates, such as "by our next quarterly appraisal" or "by November". This kind of formal assessment can be the barometer which ultimately leads to pay rises, bonuses, even promotions and should be treated as such.

By setting these targets and goals with specific time periods, you can start to measure jointly with the employee, what you'd hope they could achieve and how close they've come to attaining their goals. An employee can really feel a part of the assessment process and when you both set the goals together, it's very difficult for an employee to then say at a later date, that you were being unreasonable in how high you'd set the bar. After all, both of you will have previously set that bar together!

If you really want to make the appraisal transparent to the employee, you can actually come up with a clear marking scheme. For example you could create a series of sections such as attendance, timekeeping, development, achievements, targets met, etc. and then literally give each section a mark out of 10. 10 would be outstanding, 1 would be unacceptable. It's up to you. By the end of the appraisal this mark will then go towards a total mark, which you can compare to previous appraisals to define progress or otherwise.

Within this marking scheme you could even add in feedback from others. Any comments that have been gathered from patients, colleagues, owners and so on during the last quarter, can all be introduced into the evaluation. This will show to the employee that it's certainly not just about what you think but the opinions of all those who regularly deal with them.

The key to these appraisals are the EIGHT Ps!

1) PREPARED – have lots of information ready to introduce to the meeting.
2) POSITIVE – concentrate on what's been done well and be constructive not destructive in your feedback.
3) POLITE – be calm and in control throughout. Be reasonable, even with problem employees.
4) PLAIN – use plain English. Be very clear and concise with your communication, so the entire appraisal is unambiguous.
5) PAY ATTENTION – Listen carefully to what they have said to you. This meeting is about how they feel and how they perceive their role within the practice.
6) PERFORMANCE - this is an opportunity to fully assess how an employee has been performing.
7) PRODUCTIVE – the outcome of the meeting is that both you and the employee feel that they've been heard.

8) PROGRESS – and if all seven Ps thus far have been adhered to, then this will lead to genuine progress going forward for the employee and your relationship with them.

While there is no such thing as a one size fits all way in which to conduct staff appraisals, here's an example of how one manager conducts their one to ones:

I always start by catching up with them on anything that has being going on away from the workplace such as if a relative had been ill or if they'd recently been on holiday. I don't pry but I do show an interest and I think that always adds a personal touch to proceedings.

I will then begin to refer back to the last appraisal we had together. I effectively start where we left off by checking that the action points have all been acted upon. For example if they asked for training how it went, if they asked for a new responsibility, how they've taken to it, and so on.

Equally I will take a moment and start recollecting general observations about their contribution to the team and practice since we last got together. Constructive feedback is always important at this stage just as long as it is delivered with empathy and courtesy.

One thing I've learned over the years that one to ones with employees you've known for a long time need freshening up, so I will often conduct them away from the office at a coffee shop or even over lunch – anything to make the employee feel as though it is different to the last ones we've had together. This neutral environment can also have the effect of relaxing the individual, which can lead to a greater honesty to the session.

*In advance of my appraisals I will always ask them what **they** wish to discuss within the meeting so that the agenda is not solely based on my issues. In particular I ask them to think about how they want to proceed going forward and if there's anything they'd like to change. I always try to make this happen before we discuss my agenda.*

If I was breaking it down into a step by step how I do everything it would probably go like this:

1) *A few minutes of informal catching up – the ice breaker part of the appraisal in which I try to relax the employee. It's an opportunity to show them that you are genuinely interested in them and their lives.*
2) *The employee's agenda in which we discuss what they want to raise.*
3) *I deliver my assessment on their performance since the last get together. This is always a carefully assembled pre-prepared set of notes which I have constructed through detailed discussion with colleagues.*
4) *A point by point discussion on the action points we raised together at the end of the last meeting. Have the targets been realised and if not, where it may have gone wrong?*
5) *Create a new action plan for the next few weeks/months before the next appraisal. This has to be agreed upon by both parties and not simply an order from me. I always try to put a timescale on each action wherever possible.*
6) *Together we then assemble a brief summary of what has happened at the appraisal and all the points raised – this will ultimately form the basis of a formal sheet I put together which will summarise the one to one and which they will have to sign when it is formally typed up.*

This is not to say, of course, that feedback solely has to be reserved for these formal quarterly meetings. In truth, feedback should be a regular spontaneous occurrence. Whenever you feel it appropriate to comment on something you've noticed, do so.

Let the staff know how aware you are of everything that goes on in the practice. Give them a sense that you are interested in every aspect of it and every individual within it. It's always a good idea, after such an observation, to make a note of what you've seen, so that you can refer back to it at a late date. It gives a real sense that you are in control of your practice and there is little that escapes your notice.

As a leader you should always give praise where appropriate. Positive observations have a noticeable effect on staff. It shows not only that they are appreciated but also that you have recognised their work. It can provide a real lift to a staff member, so never underestimate its power.

Too often managers forget the impact of positive feedback and only ever seem to have a word with staff, when they've done something wrong. Don't become one of those bosses who only comments to a staff member when they have erred.

If they deserve it, let them know that they've excelled. Perhaps in earshot of other staff, so the employee concerned can feel an even greater lift from it. There's nothing like an audience when you have done well!

If you do have to criticise, then make sure that there is a constructive element. To say "that's not good enough" or "I can't believe you've done that," is like scalding a naughty child and serves only to embarrass or humiliate. The purpose of managerial criticism is not simply to point out an error but is moreover to make sure that error doesn't happen again.

A manager who calmly offers advice to an employee on how best to carry out a duty in future, is going to have a far greater impact than one who reverts to bawling out sharp criticism.

There is a golden rule when it comes to staff feedback – "praise in public, criticise in private". Managers who stick to this principle will create a much healthier atmosphere within the practice and in reality will be have a great deal more respect from the staff for adhering to this principle. After all, nobody wants to be criticised in the first place but to have that criticism conducted in front of others, will only serve to exacerbate rather than improve. It will certainly lead to a much healthier working relationship between yourself and the employee concerned, if criticism is conducted away from prying ears.

Managers, whether new to the job or seasoned veterans, will often refer to themselves as having "an open door policy". They see it as seemingly offering employees an opportunity to come and see them whenever they've an issue of concern. Sometimes, though, these are merely hollow words.

Too often an employee will pluck up the courage to consult a PM with a problem and will be met with a manager who is too busy to give it the attention the employee feels it needs. Worse still, an employee can be regularly moved on with a dismissive, "I'm too busy to deal with this right now!"

Now of course, there are occasions in which PMs are buried under a hefty workload but their response to an employee in such circumstances, can be the key to how they are perceived as managers.

The Dental Practice "Jugglers"

For example, if an employee brings to their attention something which they feel is significant, a busy PM who replies with a time at which the employee should return with the issue, is going to create a much more positive feeling to that staff member.

Imagine how much more positive an employee will feel if you reply to their problem with, *"Thanks for bringing this matter to my attention. I appreciate you doing so. I've just got this report to complete for the owner. Please could you come back at 3pm and I will have more time to deal with it properly then."*

Naturally, if you can then follow that up, by calling the employee to you as 3pm approaches, it will also give them the sense that you consider their issue an important one.

In the busy life of a PM, with so many matters to deal with and so many people demanding of your time, it is essential to make a note somewhere of the pending *"3 pm employee meeting"*. The last thing a manager wants to do in these circumstances is to forget what they've promised. To eradicate this common error, either a post-it note stuck to your computer screen, or better still, an alarm set on your mobile phone, will ensure that the employee will not be overlooked.

The extra bonus in remembering the employee in this situation is that if, by 3pm, you are still too busy to talk to them, a quick visit to the employee as 3pm nears, will at least reassure them that they've not been pushed aside. A PM who can say, *"I know I said come back at 3 but would it be okay if we push it back to 330?"* gives a much more positive feeling than the PM who simply forgets altogether.

Having spent the right amount of time coaching your employees, you will still feel the need to ensure that they are carrying out their duties effectively. While the appraisals will form a significant part of the monitoring process, an occasional check that they are fulfilling their brief can work wonders for both you and the employee.

This doesn't have to be anything dramatic; just a simple *"how are you finding the task I set you?"* offers them the chance to convey anything they need to. In most cases you will usually receive a positive *"it's fine"* response from the employee. If so, you should respond with a complementary reply such as *"That's fantastic, well done,"* and move on.

As well as reassuring you that the task you've set is being dealt with, you will be delighted with the affect that this dialogue will have had on the employee. In just a few seconds, they will feel both uplifted and assured that you've taken a genuine interest in their work, rather than leaving them to it. This will be dealt with in much greater detail in the delegation section of the book but is all part of the successful coaching process.

Conversely of course, it could well be the employee who first seeks you out for advice and as mentioned earlier in this chapter, the key is not to be dismissive. While you may be tempted to come up with a so called "quick fix" solution so that you can continue doing your work, this could well be counter- productive.

What you should ideally be striving for, is to assist them to find their own solution to the current problem; even if experience tells you how to solve their issue, it is better to simply nudge them in the right direction and allow them to figure the rest out for themselves.

This is a much more empowering strategy to adopt, allowing them to feel as though they still have ownership of the task that they were originally set. It also has the effect of allowing them to feel as though they can solve their own issues. This will hopefully reduce the number of occasions on which they will feel the need to come to you for a solution in the future. That feeling as though they've solved their own issue, is a hugely satisfying one and a situation which they will want to repeat in the future.

Earlier in the chapter we referred to the principle of "praise in public, criticise in private". Let us now extend this rule still further, into the context of being a successful coach.

This important rule actually lends itself to creating the right kind of atmosphere, which is much more conducive to excellent coaching. After all, if employees can see that the majority of your "criticism" is constructive, they will begin to understand that it is meant to be for their benefit and not to their detriment. The last thing a PM needs is to be responsible for a practice where employees are so fearful of making an error, that they will do anything to cover up their mistakes.

One of the key principles of good coaching is an acceptance that errors will be made. The key is to ensure that employees learn from them; and the best way of ensuring that, is by creating this desirable atmosphere of constructive rather than destructive criticism.

If an employee makes a mistake when first handed a new task, it is vital that a good coach adopts the right attitude. Though it is perfectly natural for a PM to feel frustrated, or even let down by the employee's failure to carry out the task correctly, how you deal with this situation, is a key indicator to how successful a coach you are.

Good coaches (and let's assume that's what you want to be), need to conceal any feelings of frustration and instead adopt calm and measured responses. While it would be ridiculous to be entirely positive about the employee's mistake, it is essential that you first try to find why the error occurred.

Good communication is the key at this point; ask them relevant questions about each step they took and try to build up a picture of where it went wrong. Once you establish when and why things started to slip, it is again absolutely crucial not to react angrily or with despair. (Even if you do feel exasperated!) Managers do sometimes have to become good actors and this is one such occasion when these "acting" skills need to come to the fore.

A good coach needs to calmly point out where this task failed and more importantly describe in detail, the correct way in which to prevent this happening again. While it is important not to come across as patronising, it is equally imperative that all the procedures are fully explained to the employee.

This detailed and measured explanation will serve two purposes; 1) it will ensure that if the employee does make the same mistake again, you will know for sure that this task is probably beyond them; 2) it will demonstrate to the employee that you are a good, patient and understanding leader who simply wants them to succeed – that is in essence, the definition of a good coach.

Another part of the coaching process is the constant measurement of employee performance. A coach needs to know how those who come under their guidance are progressing. Naturally a great deal of this will come from getting to know each individual better and knowing how determined they are to succeed or to improve themselves.

PMs will certainly have an instinct when it comes to this, particularly if they have been part of the practice for any great length of time; but even PMs who haven't been at the practice for long, will quickly sense which employees are ambitious and would welcome a challenge, against those who are quite content to stay firmly rooted on "easy street".

Whichever category you believe an employee fits into, it is still essential that you attempt to coach them, regardless of how much experience they feel they have, or how resistant they might be to embrace new ideas. In every practice, there are employees who will believe there is nothing new they need to know and nothing else they need to be taught. As a first class manager, you must not allow their stubbornness to be the decisive factor in determining whether you coach them or not. Good PMs should always try and in order to establish why they should be willing to persevere, let's look momentarily at a completely different industry.

Without good coaches in sport, individual talents would often go to waste. Coaches in a sporting arena, work off the principle that everyone can be improved. Though it is the case that those who are more willing to learn are the most likely to benefit from their work, coaches are still determined to do what they can to improve everyone, even those who are stubborn. The very best coaches in sport will often measure their own skills, by seeing whether they can make progress with even the most awkward of sportsmen and women.

A PM needs to have a similar attitude. Coaching should certainly not be restricted to just the novice who wants to acquire more skills. In reality, a hungry "newbie" is the easiest individual for a manager to work with. They are expected to make errors and will not have picked up any of the bad habits that the more experienced members of the practice may have already adopted.

Coaching a willing employee is therefore not a challenge for a PM; trying to change someone who seems to be set in their ways, most definitely is. It is worth bearing in mind that those with the most experience, are often the ones who usually have the most responsibilities. It is the case therefore, that should they consistently make basic errors, this is surely going to leave you with the biggest headaches!

In our regular dealings with PMs, we are often told that the greatest challenge they face is how to win over the *"know –it-alls"*. The actual challenge, however, is not how to win them over, but is actually how best to make sure they make *your* job as enjoyable as possible. The most cantankerous employee can remain as obnoxious and unfriendly as they like, as long as they carry out their duties in the way you want them to; and to ensure that they carry out those duties to your satisfaction, you simply *HAVE* to coach them!

Let's take a specific scenario: You've an experienced head receptionist, who has been at the practice since she left school. She was one of the principal dentist's first ever appointments. As the years have gone on she's developed a range of poor working practices; she's a clock watcher and regularly leaves the reception desk empty for tea breaks, toilet breaks and private conversations. Patients are regularly left waiting at the desk and phone calls are often unanswered. It is a situation that you know can't be allowed to continue, regardless of the number of years she's been there. As a manager you may be thinking in terms of confrontation but as a coach you should be thinking in terms of improvement.

As we've discussed before, a manager is not attempting to win a popularity contest but moreover to make the practice an efficient, professional business. In order to achieve this, they have to ensure that patients have someone to greet them whenever they arrive and someone to answer their calls when they ring. If the head receptionist is failing to meet these two basic requirements, action has to be taken and as a coach that means dedicating a period of time to advise those who work on the desk.

At this point it is essential that you think about the significant difference between pointing out what doesn't happen and describing in detail what should. The coach's role therefore is not to criticise the head receptionist but is moreover to demonstrate how an ideal reception desk should operate. This is where the smart thinking *"coach"* can demonstrate their skills.

Rather than revealing any sense of anger or annoyance, instead, introduce a range of *"ideas"* that you have devised to make the reception area a more productive place. Describe other rival practices you have seen where these ideas have worked and how positively these principles have been received by their patients.

Make sure you tell *all* the reception staff as a group and not just the problem employee and ask them to point out any problems which arise as a result of putting them into place – you are, after all, a PM they can come to whenever they have a problem.

If you feel it necessary to help with this strategy, then perhaps let the reception staff know that you are looking at all areas of the practice, not just theirs. Explain to them that you are simply trying to make the business the best it can be.

By adopting this method, though the head receptionist may not like these new ideas, she certainly couldn't accuse you of singling her out for criticism. After all, these are simply new ideas you are introducing to try to create the ideal reception area and not just a reflection of what has been happening previously.

In this scenario, the coaching does not end there of course. After a period of time in which these new ideas have been adopted, it is important for the PM to measure how effectively they have been working and equally how well the receptionists have been carrying them out.

If, for example, you have introduced a system whereby a receptionist shouldn't leave the desk unattended at ANY time, you need to check that the problem receptionist hasn't been taking advantage of her less experienced juniors; make sure she's not continually insisting the others are covering for her, as she maintains her bad habit of regularly disappearing.

In effect, it is essential that your coaching responsibilities don't end at the introduction and implementation of a new policy. As a matter of course, you should make subsequent regular visits to the reception area. You need to monitor the reception staff both collectively and individually and to better understand what is happening; and finally, if necessary, carry out some additional coaching, if these new ideas are still proving problematic. If you believe in putting something right, you have to be determined to see it through.

In reality, this kind of constant assessment and these regular attempts to seek staff improvements, are the cornerstones of good leadership. The best managers are those who understand the importance of coaching and the best coaches are those who demonstrate their commitment and perseverance to this challenge, no matter the obstacles. Always remember that the best teams will always have the best coaches as their leaders.

Chapter 6

Delegation

In our experience, PMs often seem to forget that it takes an entire team to run an effective practice and that however good they may be, or however much they'd like to, they simply can't do everything themselves. Having worked with PMs for several years, it is clear that they are some of the most talented, hard-working and reliable group of employees we've ever come across and it is often their exceptionally high standards which can sometimes prevent them from doing the one thing which would help them to perform even more effectively – and that is to delegate. Delegation is one of the first things we encourage on any of our leadership courses.

We can recount numerous tales of PMs working around the clock, seven days a week, fifty two weeks a year, in a bid to take responsibility for every aspect of the business, feeling that unless they do it themselves, it simply won't get done satisfactorily. The irony is that this attitude, though

The Dental Practice "Jugglers"

admirable in some ways, can actually have a detrimental effect on the PM's own performance.

We speak to many PMs who have actually described themselves as "control freaks"; who would rather take responsibility for every task within the practice than hand it over to someone else. One PM we coached recently believes that she's one of many:

"That was me up until the first session I worked with Alistair and Ashley at the PM club. I was one of those managers; I just did not give anything away, because I didn't trust anybody to do it. When I had handed things over in the past, I ended up having to take them back because they weren't being done at all, or they were just done so badly, that it was probably having a negative effect on the business.

After that first coaching session, I really did take on board what Ashley and Alistair had been talking about and delegating to take some of the stress away. I suppose it was really just sitting people down and saying, listen I think that you will really be good at this, that you really could help me out and the business out, if you could take this on.

Then I would sit them down and take them through it step by step; I watched them as they did it and offered coaching and support to make sure that they understood it completely. Then, as much as it broke my heart, I walked away and just let them get on with it.

I suppose it's a control thing. I suppose PMs think, I'm the be all and end all and everything has to be perfect, or it will come back on me. When you've spent so many years being a total control freak, and when you have to hand something away, it is really heart breaking. You maybe think, they'll do it better than me. Maybe I've been doing it wrong. A lot of PMs are sort of thrust into this job with no training and it's like 'off you go- go manage!' It's worrying I suppose in a way, to think that maybe someone else could do a task better than you.

I know why a PM feels like they can't let go but I think that for their own sanity, they need to look at the bigger picture. They need to ask,' is it appropriate for someone who is on a high wage to be doing a job you could be giving to someone who is straight out of school with no training?'

A PM won't be getting any job satisfaction from doing those stupid little tasks either. We thrive on the big things, like putting out a brand new marketing plan or something sizeable – that's the stuff we love doing. It's the big things which really tick our boxes. When you are doing the silly things, like recalls that a receptionist could do, you're not reaching your full potential."

Before we look more closely at the delegation process, let's take a look at the definition: *Delegation* is the assignment of any responsibility or authority to another person (normally from a manager to a subordinate) to carry out specific activities.

It is one of the core concepts of leadership. This does not mean giving up responsibility, as you still remain accountable, but moreover that the person who is delegated to, completes the task to the best of their ability. Delegation, if properly done, is **not** abdication.

Like it or not, therefore, delegation is a must; and the starting point has to be the acceptance, that by giving out some of your tasks to others, it will actually help you to be a better PM; and let's be honest, if you can become an even better version of yourself, that simply has to be incentive in itself!

The Dental Practice "Jugglers"

If we continue this adage still further and you accept that you are a good PM, then that will mean that you've conducted each aspect of your job to a high standard. That means that you've recruited good staff, coached them well and instilled into them, your own work ethic. While naturally, not every member of staff will mirror all your many qualities, there will be some employees who you feel do possess the traits necessary to be as successful as you are.

Even if you haven't been responsible for the recruitment processes at your practice, it is hard to imagine that an owner, who recognised your qualities when they appointed you, will have failed to apply those same criteria as they've assembled the team around you. A PM who believes that nobody within the practice can be trusted with any delegated tasks, should actually look at their own coaching and mentoring abilities; it is highly likely that if a PM is surrounded by a team they feel is ill equipped to take on any further responsibilities, it demonstrates they've neglected one of the cornerstones of good management – coaching.

On the assumption, therefore, that you have indeed coached well, it is time to trust your teaching abilities. There is a team of people around you, who, though busy, do have the potential to take on more responsibilities; it is now up to you to identify who they are and with what they can be trusted.

The first stage of delegation is to rely on your instincts. In your dealings with your staff, you will have seen them demonstrate certain qualities in certain areas which would make them ideal for some of the tasks with which you are presented. If an employee is empathetic, ask them to take over some of your duties which involve patient interaction;

if you've an employee who has excellent IT skills, use them to assemble your new holiday rota; an employee who has a confident phone manner, can deal with suppliers and stock orders.

Once you've established who you believe you can trust with what, you must then dedicate an appropriate amount of time to describe the task you wish for them to have. Give them plenty of detail and make sure you make them aware of any pitfalls, or even short cuts, which will make the task more comfortable.

An excellent starting point is to try to create an opportunity for them to shadow you as you conduct the task, so they can see first-hand what it entails. Let them ask questions about it and even at this initial stage, let them have a go, while you observe. The more thorough you are at this early stage, the greater the likelihood of them succeeding. It is a wonderful barometer of your own abilities as a manager, if you can see someone you've coached, then subsequently complete a task you've taught them.

One additional tip that has proven successful at this early stage of delegation, is to let the individual know why you have chosen them to take on this new responsibility. Let them know the qualities you have seen them demonstrate while performing their usual duties and perhaps even describe tasks they've previously completed which have impressed. This type of communication has a dual effect – 1) it proves to them how aware you are of the goings on in the practice. 2) It makes the employee feel special. Having heard your words, it is sure to make them want to successfully fulfil their newly delegated task.

Here's how one PM we coached sees the process of delegation:

"A lot of staff look at it as an expectation that they have to work harder. You really have to be very careful, therefore, in the way that you approach it. You have to sell it to people first.

If you just walk up and say, 'from now on I want you to do this', most people will look at it as a form of punishment. You really have to have a way of saying that this is what we've been looking into and this is why we think that this is going to work; this is what it is going to do for the business and in turn this is what it going to give to you.

Say things like, 'we think that if you can do this and help us from now on, it's going to make the business better and your job better.' Simply landing stuff on people is generally just going to get them to think that they are just being asked to do more. You really have to sell the idea, before you can get anyone engaged in it.

We have even done silly little bits and pieces where it became a competition. We sold the idea and they thought, 'yes that's great' and then suddenly one person is saying "I got 6 this week", another says "I got 7 this week". Then it became that everyone really wanted to do better, to try even harder and they actually achieved more than we'd even thought."

Once you've perfected the way in which a new responsibility is presented, it's all about coaching them and giving them the encouragement they need to succeed. It is then imperative that you leave them alone to carry out their new duty.

While it would be churlish to expect a PM not to cast

an eye over their employee as they embark on it for the first time, it is equally important to give them their feeling of independence.

There is certainly no harm in observing and gauging how they are doing but try to take stock and analyse from a distance. By all means give them feedback if you deem it necessary but make sure they know they are still in control. Let them know they have the freedom to work it out on their own.

Check in on them sporadically, not obsessively. You want to know their progress but not at the cost of them feeling that you have taken responsibility back off them. Don't feel the need to dive in with a "helping hand" at every step. Don't overanalyse each step that they've taken, as it will merely result in you adding to your burden not decreasing it, as was the main intention of delegating in the first place.

As previously mentioned, the amazing array of qualities which PMs possess is strangely the main factor which prevents them from embarking on delegation. They see themselves (usually correctly) as being exceptional employees who have the ability to take on any challenge which arises. The danger in feeling this way is that PMs can then fall into the trap of becoming overbearing within the practice - in effect control freaks! And nowhere do these traits surface more obviously than during the process of delegation.

PMs quite rightly have high standards and they equally expect similar high standards from their employees. If a PM passes on a task, they want it doing to exactly the level that they are used to reaching. This expectation often leads to them looming over employees' shoulders, checking the progress of the delegated task at every stage and in some extreme cases, grabbing the delegated task back off them as they are fearful of its failure. This defeats the entire delegation process and often results in the PM doing double the amount of work, rather than halving it!

Now for a warning! Destroying the delegation process not only increases a PMs burden but can have an extremely damaging effect on the morale in the practice. The negative impact of undermining the delegation process actually exhibits a lack of trust in your team. They will start to feel a level of incompetence, while suspecting that you may have a superiority complex. These two things together create an extremely unhealthy atmosphere. Though you had good intentions, you've actually created a significant negative.

The golden rule therefore, is to force yourself to take a step back from the delegated work. Though your temptation is to be involved, it is essential that you allow the employee to do the task without interference. Allow them the opportunity to take proper ownership of it and put the onus on them to contact you, when they require guidance. A very occasional and matter of fact, *"everything ok?"* is acceptable but only when it's part of a general sweep around the practice. The only way you will ever build up any trust with your staff, is to give them the opportunity to prove they deserve it. Given the chance, they might just surprise you.

If, having been given the chance to thrive independently, an employee makes a mess of their delegated task, this doesn't give you the opportunity to pour scorn on the whole concept of delegation. In reality, the most important thing to do is to work with them, to find out where the errors were made. It has to be stressed once again, that you ultimately want them to succeed, in order to relieve some of your excessive workload. On the assumption that you're a good judge of an individual's suitability to have been given the task in the first instance, they have to be given the chance to prove you right!

It is also worth bearing in mind, that what you consider an unsatisfactory attempt, might actually not be that bad. Try to think back to when you were first handed a new challenge – did you do as good a job at the very first attempt, as you did latterly? Remember that striving for what you consider to be perfection from an employee, is too high a standard to expect and that more often than not, *"good enough is good enough"* when it comes to a delegated task.

Equally when you aren't satisfied with the standard of a delegated task, perhaps it may be a moment to look into the mirror and not at the employee. Ask yourself this important question: *Is it possible that your coaching wasn't quite good enough and that you, yourself may have to share some of the blame for the task's failure this time?* At the risk of being repetitive, the ultimate goal is for the delegated task to be a success, so rather than give up, persevere, as the end game will ultimately be worth it.

A PM who can reflect upon a series of successfully delegated tasks, can justifiably point to it, as proof of their own excellent coaching and mentoring skills. A manager who can trust their team to carry out duties that were once theirs, is evidence of their own excellent leadership. The sense of pride in knowing that they have successfully delegated within their practice, is one of the greatest feelings a manager can experience and the amount of time successful delegation gives them to concentrate on other tasks within the practice, is worth its weight in gold. A good delegator is a good manager and the benefits are immeasurable.

We have met so many PMs who have come to us, complaining that they feel almost paralysed by the volume of work they have to contend with. Many describe how they can never switch off, of their evenings and weekends being immersed in work related issues and that their family life has been suffering as a result. They seem stressed, physically tired and mentally at breaking point and when we begin to delve into the source of their problems, it is quickly apparent that a lack of successful delegation is at its core.

Delegation is not simply advisable, it is essential and to give up on it, rather than persevere, is one of the most fundamental errors that a PM can make.

One of the most advantageous by-products of successful delegation is that it actually helps to develop new staff members, giving them the opportunity to gain extra skills which can, not only help them thrive as an individual but in the longer term can start to benefit the business. The more responsibilities that an employee has been allocated, the greater chance they will have, further down the line, of stepping up into new more responsible positions within the practice. When, either creating or replacing a departing employee, a PM only needs to look within the existing staff for an in-house promotion, it is yet another indication that the PM herself, has been operating effectively.

Though it is clear that delegation is a win-win when done appropriately, this does not mean that you can delegate just anything. To determine when delegation is most appropriate, there are five key questions you need to ask yourself:

- Is there someone else who has (or can be given) the necessary information or expertise to complete the task? Essentially is this a task that someone else can do, or is it critical that you do it yourself?
- Does the task provide an opportunity to grow and develop another person's skills?
- Is this a task that will recur, in a similar form, in the future?
- Do you have enough time to delegate the job effectively? Time must be available for adequate training, for questions and answers, for opportunities to check progress, and for rework if necessary.
- Is this a task that I should delegate? Tasks critical for long-term success (for example, recruiting the right people for your team) demand your attention alone.

If you can answer "yes" to most of the above questions, then it could well be worth delegating the task: and when you do pass on responsibility, DON'T try to analyse every single detail of what staff have to do.

When you give an employee something new to do, let them have control of it; don't feel the need to dive in with advice and guidance. Let them make decisions, mistakes if necessary before you feel the necessity to jump in. It is important to see how they learn from those mistakes and then equally how they react to making them.

Having tried to assist you in making choices over what you *can* delegate, here is a rough guide to tasks which are generally considered to be beyond delegation. Though this is by no means a definitive list, here are nine key areas which managers should consider their responsibility only:

1. **Their/the practice's vision.** Conveying a vision is the essence of leadership, so if a PM attempts to hand off the creation of a vision to someone else, they may as well be delegating away their leadership. It is, sometimes, a good idea to get others involved in the early stages of its creation but ultimately PMs must have overall approval.
2. **Hiring.** Hiring talent is one of the most important things a manager can do in order to be successful. Why would you delegate such an important process? Gathering references, doing research and gauging personalities have to be done by the PM themselves, with the final choice resting with their own personal intuition.
3. **Coaching/mentoring.** PMs simply have to be responsible for developing talent. They should take an active role in harnessing potential, teaching and guiding burgeoning talent, so that they fulfil all their promise.
4. **Discipline.** PMs have to be responsible for practice discipline. While they can call on owners for support, PMs need to step up and handle the dirty work themselves.
5. **Praise and recognition.** PMs have to be able to recognise achievement and let their staff know when they've performed their role well. In order for praise to be effective, it needs to be sincere and personal, so by definition, it has to come from the PMs themselves and not from someone else.
6. **Motivation.** It's up to the PM to be the office metronome. A positive mood and a motivational

environment come from the leader, so combine enthusiasm with optimism for the ideal mood for your practice.
7. **Reorganization.** As with many of the responsibilities on this list, getting others involved is a good thing but the PM has to oversee the changes which need to be made. Successful reorganisation can and should involve the assistance of others to proceed but the overall direction has to originate from the PM.
8. **Welcoming new staff.** When a new recruit enters the practice for the first time, it is imperative that the PM is in charge of their first tentative steps. A newbie needs to know from the outset, that you are their most important guide to a successful career at the practice.
9. **Performance appraisals.** Who else could do this better than the PM? In recent years, many PMs have begun to pass the onus of this vital task to the employees themselves, with the creation of questionnaires and forms for the individuals themselves to fill out; the theory being that a busy PM can simply sign these forms off in order to complete the process. Don't become one of those PMs who have diminished and diluted this pivotal and hugely significant duty!

Like many things in business, there is no such thing as a *"one size fits all"* when it comes to a list like this. There will be some managers who feel they have such implicit trust in an individual at the practice, that they *can* delegate some of the nine tasks above – if so, then you are the exception, not the rule, and if it works for you, continue to delegate accordingly.

One PM we coached, who previously had no dental experience prior to her appointment, actually used that fact in determining which tasks she delegates:

"Because I didn't have any dental knowledge prior to joining the practice I very quickly got into the habit of delegating tasks which have a clinical base. So I will delegate certain tasks on that basis and then oversee and manage it - but use their knowledge to carry them out. So anything behind the reception door, clinically, would be delegated to the senior nurse and then we will work closely together to ensure that everything satisfies CQC.

I share reception administration with our practice co-ordinator who is also a nurse as well. She was previously a treatment co-ordinator at another practice and we work alongside icomply; between the two of us we have separated certain areas, so that it's not all on my shoulders or hers."

In marked contrast, there are still some managers who come to us, convinced that there aren't *any* tasks that they can pass on, even if there were employees they could trust to do them. They point to the complexities involved in some, the delicate nature of others, in a bid to prove how impossible it would be, to expect another member of their team to handle it.

In such circumstances, the first thing we request is for them to take a few minutes to put together a timetable of their typical week at the practice. (*This is discussed in greater detail in Chapter 9 on Time Management.*) We break the working week into ten sections, Monday morning, Monday afternoon…..right through to Friday morning and finally Friday afternoon. In each of the ten sections we ask them to make a note of what occupied their time and roughly how long each task took.

For example, Monday morning began with a ten minute morning huddle with the staff; it was followed by a thirty minute appraisal with a staff member; there was a problem with a printer which took thirty minutes and so on….. by the end of section ten, the list of what took up their week is displayed in front of us.

The exercise which then follows is quite simply a listing of tasks which CAN and tasks which CAN'T be delegated. Within a few moments, the PM is forced to admit, that the number of tasks which could be passed on to another is significant.

As the investigation continues the number of easily delegated tasks is often overwhelming. It always amazes us how often PMs still feel they have to be the ones who have to take on simple duties such as stationery ordering, when, with minimal tuition, this can easily be handed onto someone else.

It is clear that rather than it being the case that PMs **can't** delegate, it is moreover that they **won't**; and the sooner PMs realise how pivotal successful delegation can be, the quicker they can begin to maintain a healthier work/life balance.

DON'T PROCRASTINATE – DELEGATE!

Chapter 7

Staff Underperformance

One of the most significant issues facing any manager is dealing with staff who don't meet the standards expected of them. When an employee is clearly underperforming, it can quickly have a domino effect, as another colleague is then forced to carry out additional duties to make up the short fall.

Worse still, in many cases, one underperforming employee can even lead to an increased workload across the entire practice, as their sloppiness has to be repaired and tasks repeated. One employee's failings, therefore, if left unhandled, can easily have a significant impact on office morale. It is consequently, a matter which PMs have to address and quickly.

The first challenge of course, is to make sure that you aware of the underperformance; as a proactive manager, you will hopefully have a regular system of appraisal and with it, an awareness of how each employee is performing on a day to day basis. It is equally important that you are in regular contact with senior members of staff such as the head receptionist, head nurse and indeed the dentists themselves, as you seek to obtain a full picture of each individual's conduct.

You should also be aware of any comments made by patients through direct feedback or by them filling out questionnaires. PMs should, as a matter of course, have regular conversations with patients to gauge how they feel about their journeys through the practice and during these informal discussions, they can quickly ascertain if any staff member is either excelling or underperforming.

All PMs, first and foremost, need to investigate the full facts as to why the underperformance is occurring. It's imperative you always understand the background to the recent behaviour of an individual, before determining the right course of action. A PM on our recent year long programme describes this empathetic process:

"I start off by trying to have a very close working relationship with that individual; we will have regular meetings, lots of feedback, whether positive or negative and stay in touch. All the time though, I ensure they're aware that we are going to work together to get to where they need to be.

It really depends on why they were underperforming. There could be certain outside influences that they have to deal with themselves but I can be there to support them and encourage them to ensure that they keep work and home life separate. Encouragement is also key; I ask, what can I do for you? What can we do together?"

The best tools for any PM when it comes to being aware of an underlying problem are their ears! It is imperative that, as you go about your own business within the practice, that you try to monitor dialogue throughout the building. Listen out for raised voices, office gossip, storytelling and so on, as these are often good indicators that all is not well. This is not a case of eaves dropping but moreover a sensible course of action for any manager, in determining the general smooth running, or otherwise, of the business.

Too often, PMs fall into the habit of locking themselves behind a closed office door, rarely venturing out. While a manager's workload often necessitates periods of intense administrative work, it is a mistake to simply hide yourself away. A PM needs to have a visible presence throughout the practice and even a five minute break every hour, to wander about the building, can keep everybody on their toes. This simple addition to your routine will have a powerful effect on the performance levels of the entire staff and will have the additional bonus of giving you greater opportunity to detect any unrest.

Naturally, if you've established the correct lines of communication, you may well have created an environment which allows employees to come to you with any problems they may have with other colleagues. With the number of hours spent in each other's company, occasional staff conflicts are inevitable but it is important that all employees are aware that you are the person they should consult, to resolve any difference of opinion. While sometimes these conflicts are personality clashes, it is often the case, that the catalyst has been the building resentment toward another employee's continual underperformance.

Once having become aware of an employee's shortcomings, it is then important to determine if this is a rarity, or part of an established pattern. At this initial stage you need to discover whether this underperformance is only evident in one particular task, or is a general problem across all tasks.

It is likely that an employee struggles with only a certain area of their workload, while performing to an acceptable level in their other duties. If that's the case, this is more of a coaching issue and an opportunity for a PM to work with the staff member concerned, to hone their skills in that particular sphere.

All PMs have to realise that some employees are simply not equipped to deal with certain tasks and even if they are part of the general requirements of the job, allowances have to be made for those who have certain weaknesses within their overall skillset.

An employee who is generally diligent, committed and willing, may perhaps need formal training rather than chastising. The skill of any good PM is to recognise a good employee who needs help, from a bad one whose attitude is at the core of the issue.

Having established that a staff member has been regularly performing below par due to their questionable application, it is essential to enter into dialogue with the individual concerned to ascertain their own feelings about the issue. It is quite possible that the employee isn't aware that they've been underperforming and if that's the case, it is imperative that you fully describe what is reasonably expected. This is a good time to point out the errors that have been identified and any extra work that has been carried out to rectify them.

As before, some form of assistance should then be

offered. Managers have to strive for a positive solution to any problem, whatever their hunch might be about the situation. That should initially necessitate the offer of support, in the shape of coaching or even formal training.

It is only after this method of resolution fails to yield a change in performance levels, that any further steps need to be taken. If you believe you've tried everything and that disciplinary action is the only course left to you, then consider seeking legal advice to ensure that all procedures are followed correctly.

This was how one PM we were coaching recently, has been dealing with her current staff underperformance issue:

"I've really only had to deal with this problem on one or two occasions in my career and we are in the midst of the second one at the moment. It's come at a really unfortunate time at the practice when there's been a bit of conflict. The owner had been doing a lot of one to ones to try and get everyone back on side and try to work through the issues. We thought that would be the end of it but there are quite a few people really underperforming and sitting on the internet for several hours a day.

We thought that the discussions a few weeks ago would have been enough to sort out the issue but obviously it's not. This time we are going to people and saying, listen, we have noticed that you are going onto the internet for hours a day and it's really not acceptable. They are then given a very short time to prove they are not doing it anymore.

We have decided we are bringing in positional contracts as well. Basically we will want to see certain behaviours. We know the business and things that are going to benefit the business.

We are saying to the staff, we are now putting in these key performance indicators into your contracts.

So for example, the position of the treatment co-ordinator; we are going to say to them, right, we want you to be having 20 free treatment coordinator visits every month. We want you to be asking for written testimonials – so many written testimonials and video testimonials every month. We want you to be going back through the people that we sent quotes to but never got back to us – we want you to be contacting so many of those people every month and converting them into cash.

There's very little room for them to manoeuvre from that. It seems a very harsh thing to do but we think that it's the only way to get people focused and say no I don't have room to be messing about anymore – this is a serious business. We are just in the process of rolling them out and I fully expect there to be a lot of opinions on it. I got the idea from a couple of other PMs I met, for whom it had worked really well."

For many this may seem a drastic measure but as with most issues in the workplace, there is never a one size fits all solution to staff underperformance. Our golden rule is always to try everything you possibly can through dialogue and extra personal coaching, to avoid going down a disciplinary route. Disciplinary procedures are invariably stressful and wherever possible, should only ever be considered as a last resort.

Chapter 8

Managing Upwards

Though we've spent a great deal of time describing how to manage staff, of all the vast array of different skills a PM has to work on, the one they *REALLY* need to perfect, is their ability to keep the boss happy! If the boss isn't pleased with what you are doing, you won't be there for very much longer!

In whatever field you are in, a manager is only there on the behest of those who own the business and though it is usually the most senior appointed figure, the line of command still has one step higher up; it's the owner who controls your destiny and making this relationship work, is the key to your success….or otherwise!

A PM we coached on our recent year-long programme had some fascinating observations about her practice owner, which she believes is a view shared by many PMs:

"I think that dentists and practice owners are highly intelligent people, who've been to university for many years to learn these amazing skills but I just find that at times they

have very little common sense. Maybe, perhaps, they've spent all this time learning this amazing dentistry but they've never had business training as part of that course.

They can be really difficult; they can be really fixated on tiny details; they focus on the technical details but don't look at the bigger picture.

I suppose whenever I go to speak to my principal dentist, I know I literally have a 30 second window of opportunity; it means I go with one thing at a time. There is no point trying to go in there and change the entire practice; I will just about get the attention for one thing and if I'm lucky I will get one answer back on it.

I always think about these meetings in advance. I will come up with the 20 or so reasons why and condense it to as little information as possible; I will try and get the point across as effectively as possible, in a very short amount of time.

Usually I don't find it too difficult to get the owner to buy into something, because the dentists are very focused on the patient side and the technical side. They don't really want to be involved in the business side and what they actually want, is someone who will want to come along and say, 'Ok, I have noticed that this is costing us a fortune. I have looked into this and by setting this up, it will solve our problems.'

They are then usually quite happy with that because they have a lot of trust in me to do these things. It means that they don't have to worry about it. They know that I've seen a problem, I've found a solution and I'm going to sort it out.

We've had many differences of opinion. It's really difficult and certainly for the first couple of years, I would let it get to me quite a bit. It can lead to a lot of feelings like, not being valued, that you're not reaching your full potential but then you eventually get that little bit hardened to it.

You start to say to yourself, "I've seen this one before and I know that in six months' time, they will see it from where I'm standing". You just tough it out and know that if it's not going to close the business in the next couple of months, why stress about it? Let that one go, it's going to come back in the long term and I will get what I want then."

Before we discuss the best ways of ensuring this critical relationship is a healthy one, it's essential that we first understand those above us. Let us begin with a basic premise; almost without exception, the practice owner will have invested a substantial amount of their own money into making the practice profitable.

That most likely will mean that for a number of years, the owner will have worked hard, done long hours, made sacrifices and so on; and their reward for that period of commitment was then a sizeable nest egg.

While for some in that enviable position, they may have chosen to place it in a savings account, shares, or purchased a second home by a beach somewhere, in this circumstance, they have taken the decision to invest it into a business; and anybody who sets up a business is aware, that this naturally carries with it a degree of risk. As a PM, it's important that we always try to think about this, in order to better understand the emotions of those to whom we are answerable.

No matter the circumstances of a business investment, the person who is putting their money up as collateral is effectively gambling; and while there is a significant difference between placing a bet on a horse and a business investment, the practice has no more guarantees of success, than the grey mare they've backed in the 2:30 race at Ascot!

Naturally any investor in a dental practice will have conducted a detailed investigation as they attempt to determine its chance of success but even a new owner, who takes over an already high-performing practice, can't safely foresee its long term success. There are so many factors outside of a business owner's control, that there is always an element of chance. How many of them, for example, could have foreseen the impact of the Brexit decision in 2016?

In effect, therefore, a practice owner has staked a large chunk of money on something which, not only has no guarantee of earning them a return but could in some cases be lost altogether! Imagine for a moment, the pressure that situation creates and the subsequent emotions it is likely to provoke. It should begin to make you realise why your practice owner behaves the way they do at times and why their mood can change from one day to the next.

Having begun the process of putting yourself in their shoes, it is also worth adding into the equation that while staff can be transient, clock watchers and can usually forget the job as soon as they exit the practice door, an owner remains the constant. They can never truly switch off.

It perhaps explains why we hear so many tales of PMs receiving phone calls and emails late in the evening and on their days off, from an owner who seems on the surface, to have little regard for the time at which they have tried to get in touch. In most cases, it's not that they've little respect for your life away from work but actually moreover a reflection of the fact that they are always thinking about their business. A busy practice owner is simply contacting their senior member of staff, regarding a matter they feel is significant, just as it pops into their mind.

The important thing for a PM to decide is whether they feel this is becoming too intrusive. This is something that only you, yourself can determine and consequently whether it's something you feel you have to point out to them.

This kind of discussion is never an easy one to have but it comes down to one of the core factors in determining the success of a relationship between a PM and the practice owner – communication. If you have regular and constructive dialogue, no issue should seem insurmountable.

We've spoken in detail about the significance of building strong lines of communication between yourself and your staff, so it won't come as a surprise that similar attention has to be dedicated to ensuring a healthy connection upwards too. In the same way a PM understands the need for regular contact with their employees, that same principle has to apply to the boss.

There should be, as a matter of course, regular scheduled meetings between both parties at which you need to give them a report about what's been happening since you last met with them. It is important that you deliver the positives and the negatives, as honesty and transparency are paramount. If there's one golden rule when it is comes to communication with a business owner, it is to be as straightforward as possible.

If something has gone well, tell them but don't embellish it, if something has gone wrong, don't try to conceal it; they need to know exactly how the business is running and that they can trust you to keep them fully informed. When it comes to dialogue with the owner, they don't want someone who is going to be disingenuous or worse still, dishonest.

A good manager should also take responsibility for their actions and not be inclined to blame others. Covering up is not an option, as once the truth comes out, the bond of trust between the owner and the PM will start to break down; it's this bond which is the cornerstone of a successful working relationship.

The way in which you communicate is also something to consider. Some owners want very detailed explanations, others just want headlines; some owners want a constant series of meetings, scheduled or impromptu, others are content for just occasional get-togethers. You have to decide which category your boss comes into and tailor your communication accordingly. For instance, to regularly want to meet up with a manager who is content to let you make the decisions on their behalf, may actually be counterproductive.

While it isn't always easy to do and is even less easy to teach, part of the success of your relationship with the owner, actually boils down to your understanding of their personality. If they are the type of person who needs to be regularly involved, then accept that is just the way they are; if they are the kind who rarely buts in, don't interpret it as them not being interested.

Practice owners differ enormously in their approach, from those who need to know and try to manage everything, to those who embed themselves in the surgery; those who remain aloof, to those who want to be considered just like any other employee.

We referred earlier to a PM who tried to channel her

meetings with her boss into just a quick-fire thirty second hit and how well it seemed to work. It is worth remembering that though this hurried approach worked in this instance, there will always be occasions where the matter which needs to be discussed, has to be addressed for longer. It is vital that although the personality of your owner may not ordinarily necessitate lengthy meetings, important issues have to be allocated the amount of time they deserve; the trick is to ensure that these lengthier meetings are the exception and not the rule. There is certainly not a *"one size fits all"* approach when it comes to scheduling meetings with your owner.

A PM we worked with on a recent programme, described her principal dentist as being particularly easy going and consequently a meeting with this type of owner would be very different to one with an owner who immerses themselves in facts, figures and details:

"Our principal is quite unique, in that he wants to be part of the team. He wants to be involved and wants everyone to feel as though he is on the same level. As long as he's not in surgery he wants staff to feel he is approachable at any time. We do a lot of team building, social drinks and events so that we can build relationships, in order that they feel they are comfortable enough to talk to him at any time."

By contrast, many PMs though, feel it is very difficult to challenge their owners, even if they believe that they are wrong. The key to this situation is to make sure that you handle it with both sensitivity and professionalism. Trying to offer an opinion which is different to your boss is never easy but it is important not to become sycophantic.

Owners will usually take a great deal of time to deliberate before they bring in a PM. They know that this appointment is pivotal to the success of the business and that the right manager can take a huge weight of pressure off their shoulders. They will look for many traits as they seek to employ the correct person but one thing they should definitely want, is for their PM to offer opinions.

While on the one hand, this should encourage you to offer your thoughts on an issue, it shouldn't make you feel as though you always know best, so any differences of opinion need to be handled diplomatically and not argumentatively.

When presenting a contrasting view to your owner, they will always respond much more favourably to a manger who doesn't just point out something which they believe won't work but will also offer a well-reasoned alternative instead. In other words, don't simply point out the flaws in their proposal but provide details of how your approach offers a more successful outcome; you will need good preparation, plenty of evidence and specific detail in order to achieve this without offence.

Imagine a scenario in which, when presented with a new idea for the practice, a PM says haughtily in response, *"I'm sorry, that just won't work,"* to an owner who may have spent a great deal of time working on the proposal. The negativity it creates is obvious and the damage to the relationship could be long lasting. Even an owner who you believe is wide of the mark, deserves a more respectful and dignified reaction than that.

A PM needs to adopt a much more constructive tone.

"I think you're right about this needing to be addressed but would it be possible for me to take a closer look at your proposal to see if I can make it even more effective." No practice owner could possibly be offended by that, nor could they be so headstrong as to think they shouldn't wait for the PMs assessment, before implementing the proposal. Bosses don't like to be told they are wrong but can accept it, when it's handled in the correct manner.

One word of caution – pick and choose carefully the number of occasions on which you disagree with the owner. If you habitually take an opposing stance, you aren't going to endear yourself. No matter how diplomatic you are or how courteous the tone you adopt, no business owner is going to readily accept that they are regularly wrong about their own business.

In truth, it is an extremely lucky employee who will go through their working life having never had to deal with a difficult boss. That said, it is equally the case, that not all bosses are difficult; yet there has to be an acceptance in a sometimes high pressured environment, that there will still be difficult moments which arise.

The manager/owner relationship has been equated to a marriage, with the inevitable highs and lows which accompany both "couples". From a PMs perspective, they need to have the skills necessary to manage all aspects of this emotional rainbow in order to prevent a bitter divorce!

Most owners will view the effectiveness of their PMs by the number of situations they manage successfully without their need to become involved. While there are many owners who will try to oversee every aspect of their business, they don't have the time to manage it as well, so the reassurance of knowing that their PM can handle things, is a powerful way of ensuring their approval. A PM therefore needs to demonstrate initiative and to be more proactive than reactive. One of the great ways in which a PM can demonstrate that initiative, is by presenting solutions to issues which haven't even yet become apparent.

Like any role within an organisation, a PM will have a certain list of tasks which they will be expected to perform and for many, simply meeting these requirements will be sufficient to keep an owner happy; imagine though how an owner will feel if their PM presents them with an idea to make an already well –run practice operate even more effectively!

Nobody will have as great an understanding of the workings of the practice than a PM and in this unique position they can often see areas which need tweaking. Many PMs can spot these minor inefficiencies but it's only a special few, who can take that one step further by developing ways to improve them.

A manager who can, unprompted, present a new idea to an owner in this way, will not only impress but further cement the bond between them. One of the most pleasant sentences a PM can hear is, *"I trust you to make the right decision,"* from a practice owner and it is through these kind of initiatives that this kind of trust can be securely built.

There is a well-known barometer within the business world which is used by owners to judge the qualities of a good manager – *"how often does a manager bring a solution to you, compared to the number of times they bring a problem?"* It's not hard to work out how they then use this equation to determine the quality of the manager they've appointed.

The Dental Practice "Jugglers"

You should be aware that psychology plays a major part in managing upwards. The buck stops with the practice owners, they are the ones who are responsible for paying the staff and settling all the bills and as a consequence, they will understandably feel that they should be respected and even admired. They will expect and deserve a degree of reverence; and while this does not mean that you should be afraid of them, it does mean that when they directly request you to carry out a new task, that you should endeavour to make it your top priority.

In our final chapter we discuss time management and how to prioritise the list of tasks which greet you at the start of each day – but if you usually make your boss's requirements near the top of your list, you will certainly be managing your time well. A PM who can take the pressure of his/her owner is sure to be viewed positively, so as well as managing the practice efficiently, make sure you are managing your owner just as well; or maybe, even better!

Chapter 9

Time Management

We have shown throughout the book, all the many different qualities which accumulatively create an excellent manager. We have given you a plethora of ideas and advice designed to make you the best you can be. Now we need to give you the tools to ensure that you will have the time necessary to carry out all these skills to the best of your ability.

As a PM, time is one of the most precious commodities you have. In your demanding role you are under intense pressure to achieve so much but you have only a finite amount of time in which to complete every task. If dealing with staff, CQCs, planning rotas and developing plans weren't enough, you then find yourself covering for an absent team member, answering the telephone or giving up your lunch hour, to allow a receptionist to get themselves a break.

How many times have you left work with a feeling that you only achieved a fraction of what had been on your to do list? How often have you said to yourself, "if only there was an extra hour in the day?" Well in this final chapter we're going to give you at least that extra hour back, perhaps even more! We are, in effect, going to help you re-establish your relationship with time. The principles we are going to share with you have been proven to work by other PMs who were equally willing to embrace them; so let's go on a journey to make you both more productive and as a consequence, a great deal less stressed.

There was a TV programme in the "noughties" called *'You are what you eat'* in which volunteers who wanted to lose weight and live a healthier life style, would allow the producers of the programme to document what they'd eaten in a month - they would then put all the food in a bath tub! It allowed the participants the opportunity to see for themselves what they had consumed. As you can imagine the bath tubs were full of chocolate, fast food and alcohol and it was the alarming sight of this ugly pile of food and drink which had such a powerful effect; it immediately prompted the contestants to make drastic alterations to their lifestyle.

It was designed to both shock and shame, in an attempt to force the individuals to recognise how unhealthy their diet was and that this realisation would then consequently trigger them to alter it. Those who took part demonstrated immense courage as, for many, this whole concept would have been unthinkable!

So, what has this got to do with time management? Well, have you ever done an exercise to see where your time goes in a typical week? Most haven't (probably because they didn't have the time!) but if you really want to make progress, you need first and foremost to see how you've been spending your time, where it's been wasted and the activities which have taken most of your attention.

So before we share with you the key principles of time management, we need you to initially undertake the following exercise, which we briefly touched on in Chapter 6 on Delegation:

For the next working week, please fill out a sheet and document everything that you do in 30 minute sections of your day. Detail the activity that you carried out in that half an hour, like a diary entry. Make sure you do it fully and commit to completing the sheet. We understand that it may seem like an arduous task but stick with this, be committed to it and the benefits will be far reaching.

So for example you may put – *Monday 9 to 930 – held team meeting. 930 – 10, stationery ordering and so on.*

Once you have completed this week long chart, you then need to ask yourself the following questions?
1. How many "£8 per hour jobs" did I do? (By £8 per hour jobs we mean tasks that you were undertaking, which someone new and far less experienced could easily achieve.)
2. What tasks could I have comfortably delegated to another member of the team?
3. Were there tasks that I could have eliminated altogether?

(We looked at the process of delegation in great detail earlier but its direct connection to time management should be clear.)

This exercise is designed to allow you the opportunity to understand exactly where all your time is going and by applying the 1,2,3, list above, where a great deal of your energy may have been wasted; and now armed with your list, it is time to study our tips and ideas.

Technique Number One – Make and Use Lists

Every evening before leaving the office, or perhaps prior to going to bed, assemble a "to do" list for the following day.

Once complete, prioritize the items on it in order of importance -- A, B, or C.

A - Important and urgent

B - Important but not so urgent

C. Not urgent and not that important

In the morning, start your day off by immersing yourself in a category A task. These tasks are high priority and are crucial to the success of your day. It could even include structuring a new idea for the practice, which may have a significant impact not just on yourself but on the entire staff.

If you can complete perhaps three "A tasks" in a day, you will certainly feel as though it has been a productive and highly satisfying one for you. This technique has been adopted by many of the PMs we have worked with on our year-long programme, with one of our delegates, who had been recruited from outside of dentistry, particularly pleased with its success:

"I find that taking a few minutes in the evening to review my day and go through what I've done helps. I keep a list of jobs on my phone and add an 'x' to them when they are done. I save them by week, so it allows me to review what I have done. I have tried rigid scheduling but instead I now do block

scheduling and fit my tasks into this. I also spend 10 minutes every evening planning the following day; writing the lists really helps me get a lot done in a day."

Technique Two -Block Time

PMs realise the importance of operating a so-called "open door policy" giving their staff the feeling that they are approachable at any time. However, literally having an open door for too long can have a detrimental effect on your task completion. This technique may go against the grain a little but we encourage a period of time when you effectively operate a "closed door policy"; In other words, a period of each day when you can't be interrupted and during which you can concentrate on completing a number of pressing tasks.

We recommend locking yourself away to concentrate on your to do list and look at the jobs which are important and urgent. During this quiet time, don't even answer your telephone, ignore your emails and prevent team members from disturbing you.

Ensure that you have 100% focus on the task at hand and do nothing else. In our experience, this one, above all the others has the greatest impact on your time management. It doesn't matter which period of the day you decide is best, or indeed for how long you lock yourself away but it can make a huge difference.

Although it may be challenging at first to tell your team that you cannot be disturbed, once implemented, this strategy has a real freeing effect. For one PM we coached recently, it has been a true "eureka" moment:

"I shut the office door after giving everyone 'the heads up' about it. I advise them that unless the place is burning down, I am not to be disturbed!

It gives me the time to focus on a task, so that I can get more done in a shorter amount of time. My staff are supportive and respectful of it and it's had the added advantage that they've had to deal with things independently without coming to me. This gave them the confidence to continue making their own decisions rather than keep running to me and then this means I'm not disturbed as often at other times."

Technique Three- 4 words to eliminate immediately from your vocabulary

Do you have "time vampires" that work for you? These "creatures" are team members who constantly interrupt, to ask your advice and demand an instant response: it's invariably about a trivial issue and even more frustratingly, they usually already know the answer.

There is often the temptation to give into them as you don't want to come across as rude or unreasonable; but you must ask yourself, why do these vampires come in and take your valuable time? Unfortunately, it may well be your own fault.

It is highly likely that you have trained them that to consider it okay to keep interrupting you, having never previously laid down any guidelines. There are effectively, no rules of engagement and on too many occasions you have responded to them with **'leave it with me'**, only for their request to be subsequently submerged by more pressing tasks.

If you now want to make even greater progress with your time management, then you need to eliminate those four little words from your vocabulary for good!

When faced with this very issue, American interpersonal skills expert Dale Carnegie had some excellent advice in his best-selling book *'How to stop Worrying and Start Living'*. Rather than uttering those damaging words "leave it with me" he suggests turning the whole thing on its head and instead asking *them* the following four questions:

1. What is the problem?
2. What are the causes of the problem?
3. What are the possible solutions?
4. What is the best solution?

This technique allows you to coach them and forces them to think for themselves. Let your team come up with the answers rather than you and prevent this issue adding itself to your to do list.

Technique Four- Batch the Tasks

Another idea you should consider is to batch together similar tasks and attempt to do them all at once. For example, if you need to pay several invoices, or have a number of telephone calls to make, dedicate a period of time to do all the invoice and calling in one go.

This really works well as you quickly build a rhythm to undergoing each job; this rhythm ensures you complete these tasks a great deal quicker and usually with fewer mistakes.

A PM with whom we've worked for many years describes how successfully this method has been working for her:

"I build momentum when I do tasks this way. I do them in blocks e.g. I have a block of time where I will check and answer emails; I have a block of time where I will return calls; I have a block of time where I will collate invoices etc. It means that I'm not constantly jumping about from one thing to another, things flow much better and there is a sense of 'clearing my desk'. I always write my to do list for the next day and review today's and I get a tremendously good feeling ticking off so many items in this way."

Technique Five - Minimize unplanned activities

When you completed your week long diary in the opening exercise of this chapter, did you find that you were often fitting in time for unscheduled visits by reps or were suddenly faced with impromptu meetings? If so, how much time did these meetings take and what was accomplished by the end of them?

Many PMs tell us this is a regular occurrence and contributes greatly to them falling behind in their plans for the day. If you feel the same, then you need to be more ruthless and take greater control of who you meet and when.

It's vital that you begin to ensure that these meetings are planned in advance and to try to assess what kind of benefit, if any, you are likely to gain from them. While you won't always be right in your prediction, you need to dismiss any meetings which you don't feel are going to be beneficial. Your time is precious, so don't waste it on meetings which will serve little purpose or provide any real benefit.

In reality reps exist on the basis of appointments made and ultimately orders taken – in effect they need to be meeting people like you in order to justify their salaries. What you have to decide is whether you have to see them. If, when you are contacted by a rep out of the blue and your gut feeling is that there is nothing they have to offer which will benefit your business, then tell them you're not interested. It may sound brutal but you mustn't allow yourself to give up valuable time for what will, realistically, be a pointless waste of effort.

Technique Six - Don't plan anything in peak time

One thing which can eat away at your time is the hours you spend stuck in rush hour traffic. Many PMs are also parents and as such embarking on the school run necessitates a slow, painful journey, both morning and afternoon; but wherever and whenever possible, try to avoid this unproductive occurrence.

Perhaps think about relatives or friends who can carry out one of these journeys on your behalf, or maybe set off a little sooner than you currently do, to allow you an earlier arrival time at work. Those extra few minutes here and there will all start to add up as you face your increasingly lengthy to do list.

Strategy Seven- Create a 'Not to do' list

Having spoken about a 'to do list", this final tip involves you "creating" an equally important 'not to do' list! This could be the most important list you can assemble!

When you completed your week long sheet we discussed

earlier, there will undoubtedly be a list of activities that you either should not be doing or do not enjoy doing. It's possible that these activities should have been eliminated, delegated or even outsourced.

Whatever the unwanted task is, work out a way of removing it off your list and onto the 'not to do" list instead! Watching the 'to do' list shorten, while the 'not to do" list lengthens is one of the most satisfying sights a busy manager can witness; many PMs describe this is a truly cathartic experience.

We are sure that these seven strategies will free up chunks of time from your hectic schedule and the additional time you now gain, will allow you to focus on adhering to the other ideas we have discussed throughout the book. In many cases when observing busy PMs, we've witnessed that things like coaching and mentoring have been neglected by individuals who feel swamped, by an overwhelming volume of seemingly endless tasks. They know deep down, that this is wrong but feel they have no other choice. With better time management, these pivotal managerial cornerstones can once again be afforded the commitment we all know they so desperately deserve.

Though we've dedicated several chapters to the significance of your relationships with your owners and staff, it's probably fair to say that there is actually no relationship that matters quite as much as the one which you have with "father time" – maximise this relationship and all the others are likely to be a great deal healthier!

	MONDAY	TUESDAY	WEDNESDAY	THURSDAY	FRIDAY	SATURDAY	SUNDAY
8.00-8.30							
8.30-9.00							
9.00-9.30							
9.30-10.00							
10.00-10.30							
10.30-11.00							
11.00-11.30							
11.30-12.00							
12.00-12.30							

12.30-1.00							
1.00-2.00							
2.00-2.30							
2.30-3.00							
3.00-3.30							
3.30-4.00							
4.00-4.30							
After 5.00							

Epilogue

Congratulations on getting this far and finishing the book. Believe it or not, many people who buy books like this very rarely actually read them; even fewer finish them; so well done! We hope you picked up some great ideas, are inspired and have already enjoyed some success, by implementing the tips we've suggested.

People often ask us what makes a great PM? We reply that it is not just one skill or one trait, it is a combination of doing several things well, applying good habits repeatedly and being consistent; consistency is pivotal. We are strongly of the opinion that managers are not born but they are made; they are special people who have a willingness to work on their skills and an overriding desire to constantly improve.

The following eight strategies therefore, will hopefully complement everything you've learned and motivate you to take even more action in your quest to be the best.

THE GREAT 8

1. **Be in the room**. This is a strategy we love and we are happy to give the credit to the man who convinced us of its importance. Our good friend and fellow coach Nigel Risner states that when you are in the room, be in the room. By that he means that when you are conducting a meeting, or a one to one, ensure that there are no distractions, no mobiles and that nothing gets in the way. You are in the room. The only thing that matters is that you are 100% with that person, or team. And don't simply apply this in the workplace, be the same attentive individual when you are with your family and friends.
2. **Ensure that you always apply excellent listening skills**. There are various types of listening; most listen to respond, rather than listening to understand. There is a famous phrase which should always be considered *"seek first to understand, then to be understood."* And this should apply to all our relationships. Too often when we get into an argument or disagreement, we respond without thinking, rather than with empathy. If we first do our best to really understand the other person, we've a much greater opportunity to conclude our discussion in a way which satisfies both protagonists.
3. **Have a genuine thirst for knowledge and ideas**. If you read ten pages of a personal development book a day, you will most likely get through ten such books

a year and then just think of all the knowledge you can learn and apply if you read so extensively.

(If you ever need a list of books to read, please don't hesitate to contact us.)

If you have lengthy commutes into work then why not download podcasts instead? They are an excellent way of being inspired while you're stuck at the wheel in stationary traffic! Why not try Ashley's regular podcast with Chris Barrow *'Two reds are better than one'* in which successful dental professionals discuss the key to their particular success stories?

4. **Never underestimate the knowledge which already exists within your own team.** They may well surprise you with their creativity and ideas. We often hear PMs say *'leave it with me'* when a team member approaches them with a problem. Rather than adopting that reflex response, try to get into the habit of asking them what they think. In many cases, they themselves will devise the solution which will, in turn, inspire them to think for themselves and in so doing assist in their own personal growth.

5. **Operate outside your comfort zone.** The American Life Insurance Society in the 1940s famously deployed Albert E N Gray to undertake research to find out the common denominator for success. After many years of painstaking research he concluded--- *'The secret of success of every man who has ever been successful, lies in the fact that he formed the habit of doing things that failures don't like to do."*

So try to do something every day that challenges you and forces you to operate outside your comfort zone. There is surely no better way of developing your own levels of self-confidence?

6. **Be complimentary and exhibit good manners.** You may not immediately see this as the cornerstone of success but you will be surprised how big a difference it makes. Though success can be judged on ones level of achievement, to be respected and recognised by your peers is equally significant. Simply by telling someone that they did a great job or pointing out that a fellow worker did something well, will truly inspire and uplift. As your team leaves the practice at the end of a hectic day why not thank them for their contributions, to show how much you appreciate their efforts? It can guarantee they will leave with a smile and motivate them to return the following morning in equally high spirits.

7. **Remember you are the office metronome.** The whole practice will move to the rhythm you set and its mood will reflect how you are feeling. If you are upbeat and exude positivity, there is every chance that your team will feel the same way. If you want to inspire then be inspirational.

8. **Don't procrastinate!** Too often in life we put off taking decisive action, even when we know deep down that a situation demands it. We agonise and analyse and in many cases put so much effort into thinking why something might not work, that by the time we realize it might, it is simply too late! While this certainly doesn't mean you should be

too hasty, it is always worth applying this simple question – what's the worst thing that could happen? If, in reality the consequences aren't likely to be drastic, then go for it!

So there you have it – the *"great 8"*. We hope you find they work for you as well as they do for us. Armed with all this newfound knowledge, we wish you every success and look forward to meeting you on one of our courses very soon.

HAPPY JUGGLING!!!
Ashley & Alistair

Practice Managers Club

A year-long programme for forward thinking Practice Managers who are committed to improving the profitability of their practice, enhancing their team and are SERIOUS about taking action to make a difference. If you are open to new ideas to improve your Practice, your personal development and your personal life then this is for you

In addition to networking with some very sharp people during our quarterly meetings you will develop the following skills

- Mastering the art of delegation – learn how to delegate certain aspects of your job to your team members and achieve better results
- Effective time management – get more done in the day and use your time more effectively and productively
- Creating the perfect team - learn what makes people tick, how we need to communicate with them and how to influence them to our way of thinking
- Present to groups with ease and confidence – master the skills of encouraging ideas from your team and run effective and productive meetings

- Marketing to new patients – A formula to attract new patients, which includes an A to Z of a profitable website
- Learn how to handle stress and worry both in your personal and business life

For more information please email <u>ashley@thesellingcoach.com</u> or visit ashleylatter.com

PRACTICE MANAGERS ONE DAY PROGRAMME

Wouldn't it be great if every team member did exactly what they were supposed to do, in exactly the right way? Even better, if every team member went the extra mile for the practice every day. Well, some practice owners can achieve this happy state, but it takes a great deal of focus, and some great people management skills to make it happen. One of the keys to excellent leadership is first class communication and through a series of proven techniques we work on improving self-confidence, clarity and consistency of message to enhance your relationship with staff and colleagues.

During the one day programme you will learn
- How to present to groups of people and be an inspiration to your team
- Key leadership skills, so that you can influence your team to your way of thinking and encourage them to do things willingly
- Employee engagement – the master key that unlocks performance

- A three step unique approach on how to give feedback to your team members
- How to be an outstanding listener and be able to build rapport with all your team members. Understand how they tick
- The language to use which influences people to your way of thinking
- How to improve your self-confidence and increase effectiveness of presentations to staff
- How to communicate your message concisely, clearly and with impact
- How to run problem solving meetings effectively and how to get participation from your team members, so that they too come up with the ideas themselves

For more information please email ashley@thesellingcoach.com or visit ashleylatter.com

"If you are thinking of joining the Ashley Latter Practice Managers Club then stop thinking about it and book your place. If you leave it too late and miss out, you will be kicking yourself for 12 months when you see how well your competitors, who did join the program, are doing. This is seriously the best money you will ever spend on a course.

There are so many reasons why the Practice Managers Club has been the best thing I have ever done, but the main reason is being able to sit in a room with 11 other people who know and understand exactly what it is like to be a practice manager and can relate and empathise with our worries and problems. It is such a relief to be able to bring a problem to the table that seems totally unsolvable and have 11 people offer solutions and support that will actually work. Outside the sessions our closed Facebook group gives 24hr access to pick the brains of 11 likeminded people, and find out what they are doing to stay on top. In addition to this Ashley, Alistair and the entire team are there for you throughout this amazing journey and I can honestly say I have met friends for life from this group.

Unlike every other course I've been on, Ashley, Alistair and the team do not just stand at the front of a room and preach what you should be doing. They break it all down and show you how to do it, and you could not learn from anyone better than Ashley and Alistair who have worked with, and transformed, so many practices. If you are looking for enlightenment and inspiration, then this is the course for you. Trust me, you'll have so many light-bulb moments you'll be able to light up your practice for the next decade.

As for me now, I'm doing the job I actually want to do, and my team are doing the jobs they should be doing. I'm happy because I'm not juggling a million things and actually have time to plan and do the job I love. Whilst the team are all thriving with their new responsibility and fresh outlook."
Lorraine Browne, Practice Manager at Belmore Dental Implant Clinic.

"I've joined the Practice Managers Club to meet other managers, pick their brains, learn new ideas and develop my skills as a manager as my role grows and progresses. I've taken so much from the course and it has been fantastic to work with different managers. The progress that they've made over the

sessions has been brilliant to see and I'd highly recommend it if you are looking to develop your skills as a manager and leader."
Kate Holden, Practice Manager at Sharoe Green Dental Practice

"I'm part of Ashley Latter's Practice Managers club working with like-minded practice managers throughout the year. I have really enjoyed learning new ideas which I can implement back at my practice. Over the meetings, we've discussed everything from staffing, to marketing, to management. There are a number of presenters which has made the programme thoroughly enjoyable and I'd recommend this to any practice manager thinking of joining."
Amanda Small, Practice Manager at Helens Bay Dental

"I joined the Practice Managers Club as I am fairly new to the job role (around 18 months). Before I joined, if I am honest, I was lacking in confidence and I found it difficult dealing with staffing issues and HR issues. Since I've been on this club, I have certainly grown in confidence, both presenting within the group, and back in the practice and I have been able to deal with all the issues which I previously found challenging. I would definitely recommend this club to any practice manager –experienced or not – as there is so much you can learn."
Helen Fox, Practice Manager at Marple Dental Practice

"I joined the programme in May 2017 and it's been a great investment in both time and money and I would encourage any professional Practice Manager to join the Serious Players Club which is dedicated to Practice Managers. I can honestly say it is this course that has taken a huge weight of my shoulders and I can tell you "it's liberating"!

The course has taught me to delegate and at the same time develop my team - Win Win.

I can now dedicate more time to business planning, and instead of the old daily firefighting, I now have time to do the work that really makes a difference to the practice.

I am motivated in my role to do things differently and the results are showing right through the business. Patients and our team are benefiting, patient numbers are up by 10%, treatment plan acceptance is at an all-time high and patient reviews on our website are fabulous.

I would recommend this course to any Practice Manager who want to make a difference and say to you… "Don't hesitate in taking the opportunity to enrol on this programme. Go with an open mind, learn new skills, embrace them, and use them in your everyday job. You will feel rejuvenated, motivated, you will achieve job satisfaction and a better work life balance".

Lesley Holden, Business Manager at Sharoe Green Dental Practice, Preston.

"I was slightly sceptical initially regards joining the PM Club especially with it being held in Manchester, however I am so pleased I did. I have thoroughly enjoyed working with Ashley, Alistair, and their team. I have found the course material very good, the mentoring approach excellent and working/sharing ideas with other Practice Managers extremely helpful. Each day attended exceeds my expectations and betters the one previously attended, and I love the assignments given that reinforce what has been discussed and learnt, ultimately building my knowledge.

I would thoroughly recommend anyone thinking of booking to do so and tap into Ashley and Alistair's knowledge and expertise. A great way to gain innovative ideas on how to increase patient numbers and revenue and ultimately provide exceptional customer service."

Kerry Scott, Practice Manager at Waterden Dental, Surrey.

"I've been with the practice for eight years now and worked with Ashley for about seven of those years so I have been quite involved in a lot of the things Ashley does and I know that they work. That is why when the opportunity to join this club came along, I grabbed it with no hesitation.

All the ideas and tips that have been shared has certainly helped develop my skillset as a manager and leader. Also, it has been a fantastic opportunity to work with likeminded practice managers and business managers because it can be quite a lonely job – There is nobody else in your practice who does your job role and nobody who understands what you do so to be able to have a support system around you and others in your position is definitely worthwhile and I would definitely recommend it to any practice manager"

Claire Lord, Business Manager at Southport Road Dental, Chorley.

Lightning Source UK Ltd.
Milton Keynes UK
UKHW010043260919
350451UK00002B/4/P